Small Animal Endoscopy

Editor

BOEL A. FRANSSON

VETERINARY CLINICS OF NORTH AMERICA: SMALL ANIMAL PRACTICE

www.vetsmall.theclinics.com

July 2024 • Volume 54 • Number 4

ELSEVIER

1600 John F. Kennedy Boulevard • Suite 1800 • Philadelphia, Pennsylvania, 19103-2899

http://www.vetsmall.theclinics.com

VETERINARY CLINICS OF NORTH AMERICA: SMALL ANIMAL PRACTICE Volume 54, Number 4
July 2024 ISSN 0195-5616, ISBN-13: 978-0-443-24658-6

Editor: Stacy Eastman
Developmental Editor: Varun Gopal

Veterinary Clinics of North America: Small Animal Practice (ISSN 0195-5616) is published bimonthly by Elsevier Inc., 360 Park Avenue South, New York, NY 10010-1710. Months of issue are January, March, May, July, September, and November. Business and Editorial Offices: 1600 John F. Kennedy Blvd., Ste. 1800, Philadelphia, PA 19103-2899. Customer Service Office: 3251 Riverport Lane, Maryland Heights, MO 63043. Periodicals postage paid at New York, NY and additional mailing offices. Subscription prices are $391.00 per year (domestic individuals), $100.00 per year (domestic students/residents), $503.00 per year (Canadian individuals), $544.00 per year (international individuals), $100.00 per year (Canadian students/residents), and $220.00 per year (international students/residents). For institutional access pricing please contact Customer Service via the contact information below. To receive student/resident rate, orders must be accompanied by name of affiliated institution, date of term, and the *signature* of program/residency coordinator on institution letterhead. Orders will be billed at individual rate until proof of status is received. Foreign air speed delivery is included in all *Clinics* subscription prices. All prices are subject to change without notice. **POSTMASTER:** Send address changes to *Veterinary Clinics of North America: Small Animal Practice*, Elsevier Health Sciences Division, Subscription Customer Service, 3251 Riverport Lane, Maryland Heights, MO 63043. Customer Service (orders, claims, online, change of address): Elsevier Periodicals Customer Service, Elsevier Health Sciences Division Subscription **Customer Service 3251 Riverport Lane Maryland Heights, MO 63043. Tel: 1-800-654-2452 (U.S. and Canada); 314-447-8871 (outside U.S. and Canada). Fax: 314-447-8029. E-mail: journalscustomerservice-usa@elsevier.com (for print support); journalsonlinesupport-usa@elsevier.com (for online support).**

Reprints. For copies of 100 or more of articles in this publication, please contact the Commercial Reprints Department, Elsevier Inc., 360 Park Avenue South, New York, NY 10010-1710. Tel.: 212-633-3874; Fax: 212-633-3820; E-mail: reprints@elsevier.com.

Veterinary Clinics of North America: Small Animal Practice is also published in Japanese by Inter Zoo Publishing Co., Ltd., Aoyama Crystal-Bldg 5F, 3-5-12 Kitaaoyama, Minato-ku, Tokyo 107-0061, Japan.

Veterinary Clinics of North America: Small Animal Practice is covered in *Current Contents/Agriculture, Biology and Environmental Sciences, Science Citation Index, ASCA, MEDLINE/PubMed (Index Medicus), Excerpta Medica, and BIOSIS.*

Contributors

EDITOR

BOEL A. FRANSSON, DVM, MS, PhD
Diplomate of the American College of Veterinary Surgeons; ACVS Founding Fellow MIS (Thoracoscopy, Laparoscopy), Professor, Small Animal Surgery, Department of Veterinary Clinical Sciences, College of Veterinary Medicine, Washington State University, Pullman, Washington, USA

AUTHORS

INGRID M. BALSA, MED, DVM
Diplomate of the American College of Veterinary Surgeons-Small Animal; ACVS MIS Fellow (Small Animal- Soft Tissue); Associate Professor of Small Animal Surgery, Department of Clinical Sciences, Oregon State University, Carlson College of Veterinary Medicine, Corvallis, Oregon, USA

NICOLE J. BUOTE, DVM
Diplomate of the American College of Veterinary Surgery- Small Animal; ACVS Founding Fellow Minimally Invasive Surgery (Soft Tissue), Cornell University College of Veterinary Medicine; Associate Professor, Small Animal Surgery, Ithaca, New York, USA

BOEL A. FRANSSON, DVM, MS, PhD
Diplomate of the American College of Veterinary Surgeons; ACVS Founding Fellow MIS (Thoracoscopy, Laparoscopy); Professor, Small Animal Surgery, Department of Veterinary Clinical Sciences, College of Veterinary Medicine, Washington State University, Pullman, Washington, USA

ERIN A. GIBSON, DVM
Diplomate of the American College of Veterinary Surgeons-Small Animal; Assistant Professor of Soft Tissue Minimally Invasive Surgery, Department of Clinical Sciences and Advanced Medicine, University of Pennsylvania, Matthew J. Ryan Veterinary Hospital, Philadelphia, Pennsylvania, USA

WILLIAM HAWKER, BVSc, MANZCVS
Department of Clinical Studies, Companion Animal Hospital, The Ontario Veterinary College, University of Guelph, Guelph, Canada

SARAH MARVEL, DVM, MS
Diplomate of the American College of Veterinary Surgeons-Small Animal; Assistant Professor, Small Animal Surgery, ACVS Fellow, Surgical Oncology and MIS (SA Soft Tissue), Department of Clinical Sciences, Colorado State University, Fort Collins, Colorado, USA

ERIC MONNET, DVM, PhD
Diplomate of the American College of Veterinary Surgeons; Diplomate, European College of Veterinary Surgeon; Professor, Small Animal Surgery, ACVS Founding Fellow, MIS (SA Soft Tissue), Department of Clinical Sciences, Colorado State University, Fort Collins, Colorado, USA

HEIDI PHILLIPS, VMD
Diplomate, American College of Veterinary Surgeons- Small Animal, Associate Professor of Small Animal Surgery, Department of Veterinary Clinical Medicine, University of Illinois College of Veterinary Medicine, Urbana Illinois, USA

VALERY F. SCHARF, DVM, MS
Diplomate of the American College of Veterinary Surgeons; Associate Professor of Soft Tissue and Oncologic Surgery, Department of Clinical Sciences, NC State University, Raleigh, North Carolina, USA

AMEET SINGH, DVM
Diplomate, American College of Veterinary Surgeons (Small Animal); Dallas Veterinary Surgical Center, Professor, Department of Clinical Studies, Companion Animal Hospital, The Ontario Veterinary College, University of Guelph, Guelph, Canada

CHRIS THOMSON, DVM
Diplomate of the American College of Veterinary Surgeons - Small Animal; ACVS Fellow, Surgical Oncology, Associate Surgeon, Veterinary Specialty Hospital - North County, Ethos Veterinary Health, San Marcos, California, USA

Contents

of the esophageal hiatus, as well as a pexy of the esophagus to the diaphragm and a left sided gastropexy. Outcomes with laparoscopic treatment are comparable to those performed via laparotomy.

 Video content accompanies this article at http://www.vetsmall. theclinics.com.

Laparoscopic herniorrhaphy provides a feasible minimally invasive treatment option for dogs with peritoneal-pericardial hernias with careful case selection. This article describes the techniques, instrumentation, and challenges associated with laparoscopic peritoneal-pericardial diaphragmatic hernia repair.

Minimally invasive endoscopic surgery is growing in veterinary medicine, in large part, due to the advantages associated with reduced pain, potential for decreased complications, and increased visualization of structures through magnification and illumination. With advancing technologies, we can now improve upon natural "white light" endoscopy with fluorescence-guided imaging. Near-infrared (NIR) cameras allow for real-time, high-definition visualization of vessels, anatomic structures, and perfusion. New uses of NIR technologies during laparoscopy are continuing to grow for vascular, lymphatic, and oncologic-related techniques. Limitations exist, and future efforts need to determine optimal dosing, tissue-specific fluorophores, and veterinary-specific techniques.

Intraoperative near-infrared fluorescence imaging allows for real time, non-invasive visualization of anatomic structures (blood vessels, lymphatic vessels) or diseased states (cancer, inflammation). This technique is easily adapted to thoracoscopy and has allowed for improved detection of lung tumors and other various cancers, thoracic lymphatics, and cardiothoracic vasculature.

Significant advances in veterinary minimally invasive surgeries and procedures have occurred in the past 10 years. These advances have been allowed due to continual research into optimizing working space through one-lung ventilation techniques and carbon dioxide insufflation. Additionally, minimally invasive surgery enthusiasts have joined forces with interventionalists and, in many cases, physicians to push the boundaries, minimize pain, suffering, and time away from owners with advances in a variety of procedures. Several larger multi-institutional retrospective studies on various disease processes allow veterinarians and owners to understand that minimally invasive approaches allow for outcomes comparable to traditional open surgery and, in some cases, may now be considered the standard of care in canine and feline patients.

 Video content accompanies this article at http://www.vetsmall. theclinics.com.

Idiopathic chylothorax is a challenging clinical condition historically associated with poor resolution rates following surgical intervention. Recent advances in imaging and surgical techniques have revolutionized the treatment of this disease process. Computed tomographic lymphangiography has facilitated improved surgical planning and postoperative assessment, while intraoperative use of near-infrared fluorescence imaging aids in highly accurate intraoperative thoracic duct identification. Utilizing these advancements, minimally invasive surgical techniques have been successfully developed and have been associated with considerable improvements in surgical outcomes.

Veterinary minimally invasive surgery continues to grow as a specialty. With increasing experience in this field, comes improved accessibility as well as progressive complexity of procedures performed. Advancement in technology has been both a response to the growth and a necessary driver of continued refinement of this field. Innovative research leading to advancements in surgical equipment has led to the development of novel image acquisition platforms, cannulas, smoke evacuation systems, antifog devices, instrumentation, and ligating/hemostatic devices. These innovations will be reviewed and potential clinical applications are discussed.

 Video content accompanies this article at http://www.vetsmall. theclinics.com.

This article details the rise of surgical robots in the human surgical sphere as well as their use in veterinary medicine. Sections will describe in detail the equipment required for these procedures and the advantages and disadvantages of their use. Specific attention is given to the articulated instrumentation, which affords psychomotor benefits not only for surgical precision but also for surgeon ergonomics. A discussion of the possible indications and current use of robotics in veterinary medicine and the challenges to integrating robotics is also provided.

VETERINARY CLINICS OF NORTH AMERICA: SMALL ANIMAL PRACTICE

SERIES OF RELATED INTEREST

Veterinary Clinics: Exotic Animal Practice
https://www.vetexotic.theclinics.com/
Advances in Small Animal Care
https://www.advancesinsmallanimalcare.com/

THE CLINICS ARE NOW AVAILABLE ONLINE!
Access your subscription at:
www.theclinics.com

Preface

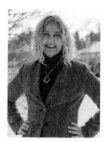

Boel A. Fransson, DVM, MS, PhD, DACVS
Editor

It is an honor to present an updated version of *Veterinary Clinics of North America: Small Animal Practice* on Endoscopy. The last issue of this topic was published in 2016, and since then, new information has been presented at a neck-breaking speed; from 2016 to today, more than 1500 articles are listed by PubMed on the theme of veterinary endoscopy.

Together with a team of coauthors who are among the most clinically progressive and scientifically productive veterinary surgeons in the world, we discuss video-assisted surgical techniques for small animals. The information in this issue is handling topics that over the last 8 years have become clinically important for practicing veterinarians. The authors present comprehensive yet concise reviews of laser-assisted endoscopic surgery to combat upper-airway obstructions, and laparoscopic correction of hiatal and peritoneal-pericardial diaphragmatic hernias. Recent advances in thoracoscopic treatments are discussed for chylothorax and other thoracoscopic techniques. The use of fluorescence to augment both laparoscopic and thoracoscopic procedures is presented in a highly accessible manner, with important information on what we currently know of dosage and timing. For the veterinarian aspiring to perform these procedures, recent advancements in surgical technology and training options are reviewed. Finally, veterinary robotic surgery is discussed and gives us all a hint on what the future holds.

This issue also aims to pique the interest among veterinarians or veterinary students who currently are not performing endoscopic surgery, hoping to convince them that acquiring the equipment and undergoing the skills training is well worth the investment in time and money. Together we can work toward decreasing surgical invasiveness while increasing the surgeon's visualization and access through endoscopy. Ultimately, endoscopy provides an opportunity to operate on small animals with reduced pain, eased recovery, and potentially better outcomes. If our pet patients were able to articulate, I am certain they will thank the veterinary profession for these advancements!

This work would not be possible without the efforts of many individuals: the coauthors who so graciously and generously shared their expertise for the benefit of us

Vet Clin Small Anim 54 (2024) ix–x
https://doi.org/10.1016/j.cvsm.2024.02.010
0195-5616/24/© 2024 Elsevier Inc. All rights reserved.

all, and the editors and staff at Elsevier in general. Specifically, Stacy Eastman, Senior Editor, and Varun Gopal, Content Development Specialist, deserve thanks. Without their insightful interest in the topic and efficient assistance, this issue would not have been possible.

With no more ado, I invite all readers to explore the exciting advances in veterinary endoscopic surgery. Happy reading!

Boel A. Fransson, DVM, MS, PhD, DACVS
Veterinary Clinical Sciences
College of Veterinary Medicine
Washington State University
Pullman, WA, USA

E-mail address:
boel_fransson@wsu.edu

New Training Options for Minimally Invasive Surgery Skills

Boel A. Fransson, DVM, PhD, DACVS*

KEYWORDS

- MIS • Veterinary training • Manual skills • Cognitive skills • Skill assessments

KEY POINTS

- New training options include a validated box training program, canine virtual reality training, physical high-fidelity models, and expanded access to training courses using animal models, but American College of Veterinary Surgeons (ACVS) surgery residents still have inconsistent access to simulation training.
- Cognitive training is equally important to manual skills training and requires cognitive task analysis. Currently, no strides have been taken toward such training for veterinary minimally invasive surgery (MIS).
- Video-based training with interceptive questions has been advantageous for cognitive MIS training.
- Script concordance testing can assess cognitive decision-making in surgery.

Minimally invasive surgery (MIS) is developing at a steady pace in veterinary medicine, with an ever increasing number of procedures added to our collective repertoire. Importantly, the complexity of more recently described surgeries is likewise increasing, with procedures such as intracorporeally sutured hiatal and peritoneal–pericardial diaphragmatic hernia, robotic cholecystectomy, and cholecystectomy in nonelective cases as a few examples. All these complex procedures have in common that they place high demands on the MIS surgeons' skills and cognitive decision-making.

Veterinary surgeons interested in performing these advanced MIS procedures have a multitude of options for practicing simulated procedures based on human anatomy and physiology. However, training modalities based on animal patients are much more limited. Unfortunately, training performed on species or simulated tissue with anatomic variations or procedural differences may not have the intended results on

Department of Veterinary Clinical Sciences, College of Veterinary Medicine, Washington State University, Pullman, WA 99164, USA
* Corresponding author. 100 Ott way, Pullman, WA 99164-6610.
E-mail address: boel_fransson@wsu.edu

Vet Clin Small Anim 54 (2024) 603–613
https://doi.org/10.1016/j.cvsm.2024.02.001
0195-5616/24/© 2024 Elsevier Inc. All rights reserved.

vetsmall.theclinics.com

skill increase. In fact, training on species different from the targeted patients may result in a falsely confident surgeon and patient safety may suffer. Therefore, ensuring appropriate validation of available training options prior to more widespread adoption is very important.

Fortunately, veterinary medicine has made progress in many areas of MIS training within the last decade. This review outlines what we have learned as a community about how to train novice MIS surgeons and what methods are available for training our future surgeons. This article also outlines general areas of training where veterinary MIS training has significant room for improvement.

TRAINING OF MINIMALLY INVASIVE SURGERY MANUAL SKILLS

Traditionally and currently, veterinary surgical skill training remains largely based on apprenticeship training in the operating room (OR). Unfortunately, it has been recognized for more than 2 decades that the apprenticeship model is unable to provide the skills needed for MIS.[1]

The manual skills needed for an MIS surgeon include ambidexterity, instrument targeting accuracy in the face of long instrument, adapting to the fulcrum effect created by the cannula, hand–eye screen coordination, and recognition of cues to provide a sense of depth despite a monocular camera view.[2,3] The OR adds further challenges such as stress, ergonomic issues, and space constraints. Therefore, these skills need to be trained until complex maneuvers such as suturing are done with ease before attempting basic or advanced procedures on the live patients. At our institution, we have noticed that if the trainee has challenges in the simulated environment, performance in the OR is not likely to be satisfactory.

Already in the early 2000s, it was noted that MIS manual skill training outside the OR was required for medical doctors (MD). A recent survey among ACVS residents indicated that residents are aware of benefits with simulation training and that there is room for improved access and the use of MIS simulation in ACVS residency programs.[4] However, as counterintuitive as it seems—the MD surgery resident training programs which have had the benefit of access to training equipment and curricula for almost 2 decades, still have problems ensuring that the residents' skills are sufficient for the OR.[5,6]

Program directors for ACVS residents need to be aware of the pitfalls and understand that buying equipment alone is not likely to result in residents with appropriate MIS skills in the OR. Aside from protected time and opportunity to use the simulator, the training needs to provide clear goals, well-validated tasks, and feedback to the trainee for appropriate skill development. For a competency-based veterinary education, assessments of the skills are also required. Therefore, parallel to the discussion about available equipment, the issue of what curricula are available and how assessments are done for each modality need to be addressed.

BOX TRAINING

Box trainers (aka video trainers) are the least expensive of the training modalities, as they are widely commercially available (**Fig. 1**) or can even simply be home made. An important advantage of these technologically basic devices is that they use real instruments that provide tactile sensation known as haptic feedback. The box trainers utilize low-cost disposable or multiuse low-fidelity tasks to train psychomotor skills. The options for tasks are indefinite, limited only by one's imagination. For example, the brilliant Japanese veterinary surgeon Hiro Kanai swears by origami folding of cranes as the best training task (Dr Kanai, personal communication,

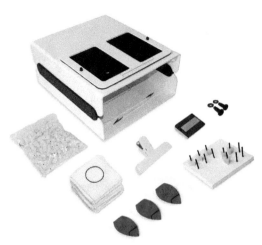

Fig. 1. Several box trainers are commercially available from a variety of manufacturers. Depicted here is the VALS box manufactured by the same company that made the box for the MD training/assessment program fundamentals in laparoscopic surgery (FLS).

2020) However, to ensure that the tasks practiced will result in actual skills utilized in the OR, validation is required. It is generally accepted that the tasks with the most solid validation to date are the ones utilized in the mandatory fundamentals of laparoscopic surgery program for MD general surgery residents. Those tasks have been adapted for veterinary use in the veterinary assessment of laparoscopic skill (VALS) program which was made available for veterinarians by the author's research team in 2017.[7] The VALS tasks (**Fig. 2**) have the distinct advantage that they provide the trainee with clear performance goals which helps self-directed trainees.

However, box training has several distinct disadvantages that educators need to be aware of. Unless the trainee is provided clear goals and landmarks for performance expectations, the training may be random and not deliberate. The trainee may focus activities on what he or she already does well because it is more fun, whereas practice of the tasks that are hard will not progress. Therefore, the resulting skill increase may not be what both trainee and educator were hoping for.

Another major hurdle for educators is the requirement for coaching and individualized expert feedback, which has been shown repeatedly to be needed for optimized training.[5,8,9] Trainees are also valuing expert feedback much higher than other types of feedback.[10,11] Unfortunately, veterinary training institutions are in general limited to very few expert MIS surgeons, and these individuals may have severe limitations on the time they can devote in the training laboratory due to the multitude of clinical, research, administrative, teaching, and other demands on their time.

Finally, the analog nature of the box trainer is not promoting easy integration between didactic learning and skill development. Box training is limited to psychomotor skill training which is only the first step of many needed to develop a competent MIS surgeon. However, for manual skill development, it is still highly valuable.[12] Importantly, box training has been clearly demonstrated to transfer skills to real surgical procedures[13] and was shown more cost-effective than virtual reality (VR) for programs with less than 10 residents,[14] a number that likely encompasses most veterinary residency programs.

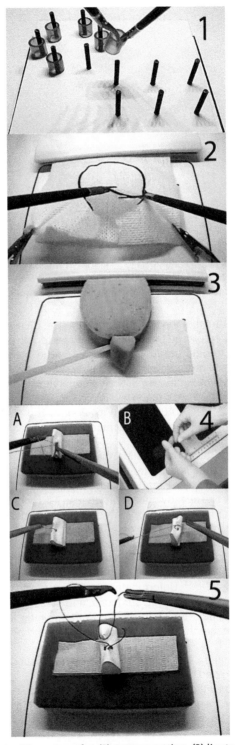

Fig. 2. The 5 VALS tasks: (1) peg transfer, (2) pattern cutting, (3) ligature loop placement, (4) A–D extracorporeal suture, and (5) intracorporeal suture.

VIRTUAL REALITY TRAINERS

The development of VR MIS training (**Fig. 3**) has provided additional opportunities for surgical educators. These highly technologically advanced training modalities carry many advantages:

- Unlimited practice: As the virtual environment requires no disposable materials, the training laboratory is easier to manage, and trainees can be allowed unlimited practice with little need for laboratory management.
- Availability of not only basic manual skill training but also surgical procedure training. Many VR trainers provide realistic "complications" such as hemorrhage, bruising, or leakage from bile duct in response to errors in technique.
- Easy integration of tutorials that can break down procedures into tasks and not only provide manual but also cognitive training.
- Realistic VR training is more exciting for surgical trainees compared to low-fidelity box training. The "fun factor" provides additional motivation for training.
- Integrated feedback in the form of motion metrics and report on errors. These are often compared to expert performance, giving the trainee perspective on their performance.
- Documented transfer of simulation-trained skills to the OR.[13]

Veterinary surgical educators also need to be aware of the disadvantages of these advanced training machines. The most problematic is likely that most surgical procedures are modeled on human anatomy and functions. This brings validity into focus, because as mentioned earlier, training surgery on the "wrong" species may not lead to safer surgeons and in worst case scenario could lead to misinformed or overconfident surgeons. Paired with the other main disadvantage which is the cost of trainer and software modules, one could argue that paying a lot and only be able to utilize the basic skill portion because surgical procedure lacks validity, is not well spent funding. In fact, the high cost of VR training was an issue raised in a recent systematic review questioning whether VR training really should be the main training modality in MD surgical training or not?[15] Currently, one of the most common and comprehensive surgery resident curricula in the United States, the American College of Surgeons/ Association of Program Directors in Surgery (ACS/APDS) national skill curriculum, is not requiring VR training with cost as a stated reason.[16,17]

However, for veterinary surgery training, validated VR simulation would be extremely valuable due to the previously mentioned relative paucity of MIS experts

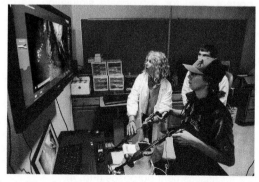

Fig. 3. Virtual reality training has the unique feature of providing unlimited surgical procedure training and automated performance assessment. However, validation for veterinary use is only beginning currently.

at many institutions. The lack of experts for feedback and assessments of veterinary trainees makes it even more urgent to have detailed training available that can combine cognitive with manual skill training. Furthermore, VR provides surgical procedures training which is highly advantageous and not readily accessible in other modalities. Surgical procedure practice in animal models is ridden with ethical, availability, and cost concerns. For the veterinary trainee who needs to progress from basic manual skills through basic surgical procedures onto advanced surgical procedures, VR training may, in the future, become the most effective training modality. However, this notion assumes that veterinary-specific training becomes available, which also needs to be validated to ensure that the training indeed leads to the intended skill development and ultimately to safer surgeons.

Recently, one of the main manufacturers of VR surgery simulators, Surgical Science (previously Simbionix), collaborated with Swedish veterinarians funded by The Greater Stockholm Veterinary Care Foundation, to develop VR training specifically for veterinarians. Thus, a VR-simulated canine laparoscopic ovariectomy model has been made available by this company. Also, the same company reached out to American diplomates of the ACVS and initiated a collaborative effort with the author to develop a curriculum for canine cholecystectomy which was made available 2022. The cholecystectomy curriculum utilizes human anatomy in the simulated surgical procedure, but the tutorials and procedure instructions were canine-specific. Further collaborative efforts with this company are currently underway and will hopefully result in additional curricula development useful for veterinary trainees.

PHYSICAL MODELS FOR SIMULATED SURGICAL PROCEDURES

Surgical procedure training can also be performed by the use of anatomically correct models, so-called high-fidelity models. Over the last 20 years, such models have become a billion-dollar industry on the MD training side. These models utilize regular surgical instrumentation and a box trainer and are thus highly accessible for many training laboratories. Currently, the main limitation is the lack of high-fidelity models of veterinary patients. To the author's knowledge, no physical models with canine or equine anatomy suitable for MIS training are currently commercially available.

Our research team investigated the feasibility and validity of custom-made models for ovariectomy in dogs[18] and horses.[19] These models were cost-effective but require a dedicated model maker for the time-consuming multistep procedure of creating these silicone models. Also, in the author's opinion, basic procedures such as ovariectomy are probably a less important need for appropriate simulation, as compared to more advanced procedures associated with a higher risk for morbidity such as adrenalectomy or cholecystectomy. Such procedures require high precision and good anatomic knowledge, and therefore, species-specific models are required. For cholecystectomy, there is some overlap between canine and human surgery, but there are still important differences in surgical technique between the 2, making specific instruction necessary if such human models are used to train veterinary surgeons. Also, for training purposes such models could become expensive. The most cost-effective model to date is likely a laparoscopic cholecystectomy (LC) model (Simulab, Seattle, WA) where the liver model costs less than $700 and each disposable gallbladder approximately $50 each (October 2023). However, at our institution, we are still unable to provide unlimited practice on such simulated tissue due to cost reasons. Instead, use of these models is perhaps more feasible for assessment purposes (**Fig. 4**).

Regardless, educators need to be prepared to provide detailed instructions on surgical techniques and dedicate time for individual feed-back if using physical models

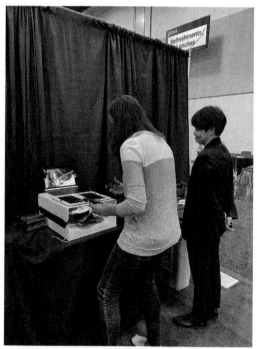

Fig. 4. High-fidelity physical models may become increasingly used in veterinary MIS training, but prior to widespread use validation is required. Here, an ACVS MIS specialist is participating in a validation study of a cholecystectomy model.

for training purposes. Currently, there appears to be a paucity of curricula available for physical model training.

SHORT COURSES ON ANIMAL MODELS

A very important step in the training of MIS surgeons is short-course training in animal models. These give important hands-on training in cadavers or live animals and are arranged by several institutions worldwide. In the author's opinion, the trainee benefits from having practiced the basic psychomotor skills before work in these cadaver or live animal models. That way the trainee could focus on the skills not well trained in basic simulation such as laparoscopic entry and performance of the actual surgical procedures without being limited by basic skill shortcomings. Many of these courses are offering simulation training as part of the curriculum, which can serve as a great introduction. However, gaining and retaining the laparoscopic skills discussed earlier requires distributed practice over longer time than a short course can offer. Importantly, a period of rest between training sessions is also necessary to provide cerebral integration and thus retention of the skills.

TRAINING OF COGNITIVE DECISION-MAKING IN MINIMALLY INVASIVE SURGERY

Traditionally, most veterinary surgical cognitive training has been taking place in the OR. Through first assisting the experienced surgeon, and later performing surgery under supervision, the resident learns the steps of the procedure and to identify relevant anatomic structures. However, this learning is dependent on how actively the resident is paying attention, especially during the important assistant stage. Also, knowledge of possible complications during each step of the procedure is important to minimize risk for errors. These may not always be apparent to the resident watching or operating under the watchful eye of an experienced surgeon. Thus, depending on the attention, working memory, memorized theoretic knowledge, and multitasking ability, the resident may or may not gain the required cognitive skills through the traditional approach. Surgeons can improve the residents' learning by didactic communication in the OR, but such training may be limited by individual variation, is time-consuming, and sometimes hard to pair with the mental load of performing surgery in live patients. Some of these limitations were demonstrated in LCs performed by residents overseen by surgeons, where less than half of the decision-making teaching points were taking place.[20] In contrast, 61% of technical teaching points were observed,[20] showing that attending surgeons may tend to focus more on teaching technical performance and less on decision-making. Unfortunately, the assumption that high level of technical skills predict the ability to perform safe surgery was challenged in a study demonstrating that most surgical errors were caused by judgment errors and vigilance or memory failures.[21]

Along with the shift from traditional to competency-based medical education, it has become more obvious that cognitive training is equally important to manual skill training. Consequently, the acquisition of cognitive competencies in MIS has recently become an active area of research. It has become apparent that the cognitive and manual skill competence is different and that specific training of the former is needed.[22] Training on separate cholecystectomy tasks on a VR simulator combined manual and cognitive training, but viewing a high-quality educational video was more effectively teaching cognitive competency.[22] Active participation ensured by interceptive questions during video-based training showed better LC performance in the OR, compared video to watching without questions.[23] An individual's perception of key elements relates to function in the complex situations such as surgery. This perception, termed situational awareness,[22,24] is related to the ability of accurate decision-making.[24] A systematic review found that simulation-based MIS surgical team crisis training is an effective way of assessing residents' situational awareness.[24] More novel methods for training situation awareness in MIS include serious gaming[25] and mental skill training,[26–28] in addition to previously mentioned surgical video-based training.

Regardless of training methods, teaching cognitive skills require analysis of critical decisions needed for optimal surgical performance, that is, cognitive task analysis.[29,30] This analysis breaks procedures down into "microsteps" used to reflect surgeon perceptions, assessments, and decisions, that is, surgeon cognition. Cognitive task analysis has recently been used in an attempt to improve MIS procedure safety.[30] MIS procedures do entail problems that do not always have straightforward algorithmic solutions. They require knowledge and insights that are hard to evaluate, have no one single correct answer, and are revealed only in authentic situations.[31] Experienced surgeons have developed complex networks of knowledge that are fitted to the case handling and surgical tasks, and these networks have been named scripts. A relatively new assessment tool has been developed for such clinical expertise, the script concordance test,[31] which has been evaluated for clinical competency examination also in veterinary medicine.[32,33] Recently, a cognitive task analysis was performed to define the difficult task of intracorporeal suturing, and a Video-based script concordance test validated after assessing experts and inexperienced surgeons.[34] Similar methods could likely improve cognitive training also for ACVS residents, who may experience inconsistent case load or lack of MIS expertise at their training institutions. Unfortunately, major limiting factor in the development of both cognitive task analysis and script concordance testing is that both are time-consuming to create. To ensure that the cognitive training captures true clinical MIS competence, both task analysis and script development require participation of experts. Paired with the current relative shortage of veterinary MIS experts, it is uncertain if and when Video-based cognitive training will be fully available for all ACVS residents.

LOOKING TO THE FUTURE: MINIMALLY INVASIVE SURGERY SURGICAL PROCEDURE SKILL ASSESSMENT

For all competency-based training, assessments are needed to verify that competence has been achieved. When assessing surgical skills directly in the OR, several practical challenges arise, but MIS carries an advantage in that the surgical procedure is video based. Thus, video-based assessments are theoretically readily available for assessing technical skills. Such assessments have many advantages such as assessor blinding which may remove bias concerns and provide convenience and flexibility as compared to real-time direct assessments.[35] However, the assessments are time-consuming and may lead to assessment burn-out by both assessors and assesses.[10] Currently, work is underway to capture artificial intelligence (AI) to accurately assess video-based performance,[36] which in the future may at least relieve MIS surgeons from some of the time-consuming task of assessing trainee performance. In addition, AI may become available as a quality assurance tool and may, in the future, even be able to help surgeons in real-time by providing annotation and decision support.

DISCLOSURE

The author is the developer of the veterinary assessment of laparoscopic skills, the VALS program. This program provides laparoscopic skill training and certifying assessment of basic laparoscopic skills and is run as a recharge operation without financial rewards to the author. The equipment for VALS is made commercially available through Limbs and Things Inc, and no royalty on sales are extended to the author. The author also collaborates with Surgical Science Inc, to provide veterinary-specific virtual reality training curricula that are commercially available. However, the author is not receiving any financial or other royalties from sales.

REFERENCES

1. Aggarwal R, Moorthy K, Darzi A. Laparoscopic skills training and assessment. Br J Surg 2004;91:1549–58.
2. Derossis AM, Fried GM, Abrahamowicz M, et al. Development of a model for training and evaluation of laparoscopic skills. Am J Surg 1998;175:482–7.
3. Rosser JC Jr, Rosser LE, Savalgi RS. Objective evaluation of a laparoscopic surgical skill program for residents and senior surgeons. Arch Surg 1998;133: 657–61.
4. Balsa IM, Giuffrida MA, Culp WTN, et al. Perceptions and experience of veterinary surgery residents with minimally invasive surgery simulation training. Vet Surg 2020;49(Suppl 1):O21–7.
5. Enani G, Watanabe Y, McKendy KM, et al. What are the Training Gaps for Acquiring Laparoscopic Suturing Skills? J Surg Educ 2017;74:656–62.

6. Schijven MP, Bemelman WA. Problems and pitfalls in modern competency-based laparoscopic training. Surg Endosc 2011;25:2159–63.

7. Fransson B.A., VALS, 2017, Available at: https://valsprogram.org/. Accessed March 7, 2024.

8. Porte MC, Xeroulis G, Reznick RK, et al. Verbal feedback from an expert is more effective than self-accessed feedback about motion efficiency in learning new surgical skills. Am J Surg 2007;193:105–10.

9. Palter VN, Grantcharov TP. Individualized deliberate practice on a virtual reality simulator improves technical performance of surgical novices in the operating room: a randomized controlled trial. Ann Surg 2014;259:443–8.

10. Axelrod C, Walker M, Swift B, et al. What is the Role of Video-Based Assessment of Laparoscopic Surgical Skill in Residency Training? A Qualitative Study of Trainee and Faculty Perspectives. J Obstet Gynaecol Can 2023;45:486–8.

11. Lovasik BP, Fay KT, Patel A, et al. Development of a laparoscopic surgical skills simulation curriculum: Enhancing resident training through directed coaching and closed-loop feedback. Surgery 2022;171:897–903.

12. Botden SM, Torab F, Buzink SN, et al. The importance of haptic feedback in laparoscopic suturing training and the additive value of virtual reality simulation. Surg Endosc 2008;22:1214–22.

13. Dawe SR, Windsor JA, Broeders JA, et al. A systematic review of surgical skills transfer after simulation-based training: laparoscopic cholecystectomy and endoscopy. Ann Surg 2014;259:236–48.

14. Orzech N, Palter VN, Reznick RK, et al. A comparison of 2 ex vivo training curricula for advanced laparoscopic skills: a randomized controlled trial. Ann Surg 2012;255:833–9.

15. Jin C, Dai L, Wang T. The application of virtual reality in the training of laparoscopic surgery: A systematic review and meta-analysis. Int J Surg 2021;87:105859.

16. Jogerst KM, Eurboonyanun C, Park YS, et al. Implementation of the ACS/APDS Resident Skills Curriculum reveals a need for rater training: An analysis using generalizability theory. Am J Surg 2021;222:541–8.

17. Scott DJ, Dunnington GL. The new ACS/APDS Skills Curriculum: moving the learning curve out of the operating room. J Gastrointest Surg 2008;12:213–21.

18. Chen CY, Elarbi M, Ragle CA, et al. Development and evaluation of a high-fidelity canine laparoscopic ovariectomy model for surgical simulation training and testing. J Am Vet Med Assoc 2019;254:113–23.

19. Elarbi MM, Ragle CA, Fransson BA, et al. Face, construct, and concurrent validity of a simulation model for laparoscopic ovariectomy in standing horses. J Am Vet Med Assoc 2018;253:92–100.

20. Pernar LI, Peyre SE, Hasson RM, et al. Exploring the Content of Intraoperative Teaching. J Surg Educ 2016;73:79–84.

21. Rogers SO Jr, Gawande AA, Kwaan M, et al. Analysis of surgical errors in closed malpractice claims at 4 liability insurers. Surgery 2006;140:25–33.

22. Yang C, Sander F, Helmert JR, et al. Cognitive and motor skill competence are different: Results from a prospective randomized trial using virtual reality simulator and educational video in laparoscopic cholecystectomy. Surgeon 2023;21:78–84.

23. Kowalewski KF, Seifert L, Kohlhas L, et al. Video-based training of situation awareness enhances minimally invasive surgical performance: a randomized controlled trial. Surg Endosc 2023;37:4962–73.

24. Graafland M, Schraagen JM, Boermeester MA, et al. Training situational awareness to reduce surgical errors in the operating room. Br J Surg 2015;102:16–23.
25. Graafland M, Bemelman WA, Schijven MP. Appraisal of face and content validity of a serious game improving situational awareness in surgical training. J Laparoendosc Adv Surg Tech 2015;25:43–9.
26. Anton NE, Beane J, Yurco AM, et al. Mental skills training effectively minimizes operative performance deterioration under stressful conditions: Results of a randomized controlled study. Am J Surg 2018;215:214–21.
27. Anton NE, Mizota T, Whiteside JA, et al. Mental skills training limits the decay in operative technical skill under stressful conditions: Results of a multisite, randomized controlled study. Surgery 2019;165:1059–64.
28. Anton NE, Bean EA, Myers E, et al. Optimizing learner engagement during mental skills training: A pilot study of small group vs. individualized training. Am J Surg 2020;219:335–9.
29. Craig C, Klein MI, Griswold J, et al. Using cognitive task analysis to identify critical decisions in the laparoscopic environment. Hum Factors 2012;54:1025–39.
30. Villarreal ME, Rothwell C, Huang E. Uncovering patient safety considerations in laparoscopic cholecystectomy using cognitive task analysis. Surg Endosc 2023;37:3921–5.
31. Charlin B, Roy L, Brailovsky C, et al. The Script Concordance test: a tool to assess the reflective clinician. Teach Learn Med 2000;12:189–95.
32. Cobb KA, Brown G, Hammond R, et al. Students' perceptions of the Script Concordance Test and its impact on their learning behavior: a mixed methods study. J Vet Med Educ 2015;42:45–52.
33. Tayce JD, Saunders AB. The Use of a Modified Script Concordance Test in Clinical Rounds to Foster and Assess Clinical Reasoning Skills. J Vet Med Educ 2022; 49:556–9.
34. Enani G, Vassiliou M, Kaneva P, et al. A Video-Based Assessment Tool to Measure Intraoperative Laparoscopic Suturing Using a Modified Script Concordance Methodology. J Surg Educ 2023;80:1005–11.
35. McQueen S, McKinnon V, VanderBeek L, et al. Video-Based Assessment in Surgical Education: A Scoping Review. J Surg Educ 2019;76:1645–54.
36. Korndorffer JR Jr, Hawn MT, Spain DA, et al. Situating Artificial Intelligence in Surgery: A Focus on Disease Severity. Ann Surg 2020;272:523–8.

Laser-Assisted Turbinectomy in Dogs

Heidi Phillips, VMD*

KEYWORDS

- Brachycephalic obstructive airway syndrome • Nasal conchae
- Rostral and caudal aberrant turbinates • Mucosal contact • Diode laser

KEY POINTS

- Primary respiratory components of brachycephalic obstructive airway syndrome (BOAS) were historically thought to only include stenotic nares, elongated soft palate, and hypoplastic trachea. It is now known that intranasal obstructions can contribute substantially to upper airway resistance. Recently identified primary components of brachycephaly include nasal vestibular stenosis, hypertrophic nasal turbinates causing increased points of mucosal contact, and aberrant rostral and caudal nasal turbinates causing intranasal obstruction.
- Laser-assisted turbinectomy is a novel endoscopic-assisted procedure that utilizes diode laser light to safely dissect and remove aberrant turbinates as well as sculpt hypertrophic turbinates to achieve turbinate volume reduction. Its use, together with other components of a modified multi-level airway surgery, has resulted in long-term airway patency; improved respiratory functional grading scores, brachycephalic obstructive airway syndrome indices, and exercise and heat tolerance; decreased airway sounds; near complete amelioration of sleep disorders; and a significant reduction in life-threatening events such as collapse and choking.
- Regrowth of turbinates to the point of obstruction results in approximately 16% of dogs following the laser-assisted turbinectomy (LATE) procedure, and the pathoetiology of conchal regrowth is not completely understood. It is recommended to remove only those conchal lamellae causing obstruction of the ventral conducting airway to preserve conchal function and prevent compensatory responses to alterations in airflow which may result in recurrence of intranasal obstruction.
- Research is ongoing to identify criteria in all brachycephalic breeds to determine which patients would benefit most from LATE.

 Video content accompanies this article at http://www.vetsmall.theclinics.com.

INTRODUCTION

Clinically and morphometrically, dogs have historically been classified according to their cranial proportions into 3 groups; brachycephalic dogs have short and wide

Department of Veterinary Clinical Medicine, Small Animal Surgery, University of Illinois College of Veterinary Medicine, 1008 West Hazelwood Drive, Urbana, IL 61802, USA
* Corresponding author.
E-mail address: philli@illinois.edu

Vet Clin Small Anim 54 (2024) 615–636
https://doi.org/10.1016/j.cvsm.2024.02.002
0195-5616/24/© 2024 Elsevier Inc. All rights reserved.

skulls, dolichocephalic dogs have long and narrow skull conformation, and mesaticephalic dogs have skull shape and size of intermediate proportions.[1]

Brachycephalic dogs are the product of artificial selection through breeding for an increasingly severe, pedomorphic, or "baby-faced," conformation as a breed standard[1]; breeds include the pug, French bulldog, English bulldog, Japanese chin, Boston terrier, Pekingese, Shih tzu, Cavalier King Charles Spaniel, Dogue de Bordeaux, Bullmastiff, and others.[2–7] A skull length to skull width ratio greater than 0.81[1,8] results from local chondrodysplasia, with the skull length measured as the distance from the prosthion to the inion and the skull width as the greatest distance between the right and left zygomatic arches.[8,9] Chondrodystrophy of the axial skeleton is focused on the middle of the face, producing facial shortening that affects the maxilla more than the mandible and creates a profound underbite, wide eye position, and variably flat nose.[1] Congenital and acquired deformities result from this craniofacial bony shortening without a concomitant reduction in the volume of nasopharyngeal and oropharyngeal soft tissues.[2,5]

BRACHYCEPHALIC OBSTRUCTIVE AIRWAY SYNDROME

Brachycephalic obstructive airway syndrome (BOAS) is a chronic, debilitating, and potentially fatal condition of brachycephalic dogs.[2,4–7] Despite the known encumbrances imposed upon the brachycephalic animal, demand for these pets is presently at its highest in decades.[1,3] Registration of brachycephalic breeds skyrocketed in recent years in the United Kingdom with registration of French bulldogs increasing 15 fold from 2200 in 2010 to over 33,000 in 2020.[10] Regarding the American Kennel Club, French and English bulldogs were in the top 10 registered breeds from 2014 to 2019, and since that time the French bulldog has risen to be the most popular registered breed.[3,5,11–13] Recently, a French bulldog was also the Non-Sporting Group Champion and won Best in Show at the 2022 Westminster Kennel Club Dog Show, evidence of pervading enthusiasm for the breed standard. The author has also recently described characteristics of a feline brachycephalic syndrome.[14,15] Brachycephalic feline breeds include the Persian, Himalayan, Burmese, Scottish fold, and exotic shorthair. While ownership of purebred cats is less common than ownership of purebred dogs, brachycephalic feline breeds are also very popular pets, with exotic shorthair and Persian cats ranking among the 4 most popular cat breeds registered with the Cat Fanciers' Association since 2012.[16]

A focus on extreme brachycephaly has led to numerous morphologic craniofacial changes affecting the nose, hard and soft palates, dentition, ear canals and middle ear, orbits and globes, tongue, and larynx, with potential for significant physiologic impact on both dogs and cats. For example, rostrocaudal shortening and laterolateral widening of the maxillary and palatine bones creates a more club-shaped hard palate in dogs, causes extreme foreshortening of the nose, and alters dentition.[1] Severe discrepancy between bony and soft tissue reduction leads to either relative hypertrophy or true hyperplasia of the nasal folds; the tongue; and the oral and nasal mucosa, muscle, and glands of the soft palate, but relative hypoplasia of other tissues such as the trachea.[1,17,18] These tissues are among the primary anatomic abnormalities contributing to BOAS.[1,6,7,19,20] Respiratory clinical signs predominate in dogs affected with BOAS, and acute signs can be exacerbated by obesity or stressful situations such as overheating, excitement, or exercise.[3,21] Signs range from mild to severe and include snoring or stertor, coughing, stridor, inspiratory dyspnea, difficulty eating, exercise intolerance, cyanosis, collapse, syncope, and death.[5,22–24] Primary respiratory components of BOAS were historically thought to only include stenotic nares, elongated soft palate, and hypoplastic trachea, diagnosed in 58% to 85%, 62% to 100%, and 13% of brachycephalic dogs, respectively.[11,17,22,25] These were addressed surgically when possible by traditional multi-level upper airway surgery (TMS) including resection alaplasty of the alar wing and cut-and-sew staphylectomy or staphylectomy using a bipolar, electrothermal, vessel-sealing device (Ligasure).[2,26–32] These traditional surgeries, variably performed and combined with resection of the everted mucosa of the laryngeal ventricles when indicated have resulted in some success.[22,33–36] However, persistence or recurrence of clinical signs is not uncommonly reported.[17,37] Continued selection for an increasingly flat face and the rise in popularity of extreme brachycephalic breeds have resulted in less successful outcomes with traditional surgery, more desperate need for accurate understanding of the problems of brachycephaly, and more focused research on these breeds.[7,13,17,38,39]

While airflow through the nasal passages reportedly accounts for nearly 80% of total airflow resistance in normal dogs, nasal resistance in brachycephalic dogs was previously attributed wholly to stenosis at the external nares.[11,32,40] However, in 2010, Lippert, Oechtering, and others showed with impulse oscillometry for the first time that brachycephalic dogs have increased *intranasal* resistance.[41] As a 50% reduction in radius results in a 16-fold increase in flow resistance, a decrease in any dimension of the nasal vestibule or intranasal passages would increase upper airway resistance in brachycephalic breeds significantly compared to non-brachycephalic dogs.[6,42,43] Yet despite the foreshortened nose being the most prominent feature of brachycephaly, traditional classifications and treatments of BOAS failed to identify or address obstructions within the intranasal airway, from the nasal vestibule to the nasal cavity to the nasopharyngeal meatus.[17,18,21,32]

INTRANASAL OBSTRUCTIONS IN BRACHYCEPHALIC OBSTRUCTIVE AIRWAY SYNDROME

Beginning in 2010 in a series of presentations and publications, Oechtering and others systematically offered evidence that, compared to normocephalic dogs, brachycephalic dogs have 1) crowded, hypertrophic nasal turbinates causing increased points of mucosal contact amongst intranasal structures,[32] 2) aberrant rostral and caudal nasopharyngeal turbinates causing obstruction of the conducting intranasal and nasopharyngeal airways,[17,21] and 3) interference with airflow at the level of the nasal vestibule due to a rigid, immobile alar fold (**Fig. 1**).[44,45] These newly uncovered primary anatomic anomalies comprise sites of moderate to severe, fixed intranasal obstruction that plague many dogs with BOAS, especially pugs, French bulldogs, and English bulldogs.[6,7,12,17,21,32,44–46]

Secondary abnormalities result from chronically increased resistance to airflow and include enlarged, hypertrophic, and everted tonsils; everted mucosa of the laryngeal ventricles; laryngeal and pharyngeal mucosal edema; nasopharyngeal mucosal hyperplasia; and laryngeal collapse (Video 1).[3,6,11,32,42,47–49] Brachycephaly has also been implicated in gastrointestinal disorders including regurgitation, vomiting, gastritis, duodenitis, hiatal hernia, and aspiration pneumonia; sleep disorders including sleep apnea; cardiopulmonary disorders including hypoxemia, hypercapnea, tracheal and bronchial collapse, polycythemia, heat stroke, and hypertension; and neoplastic disorders such as chemodectoma.[22,23,25,34,42,49] Additionally, sleep apnea in brachycephalic dogs may be linked to macroglossia, the accumulation of fat at the base of the tongue, and the development of systemic hypertension, as in people (**Fig. 2**).[5,19,20,25] It has been the author's experience that clinical signs of sleep apnea,

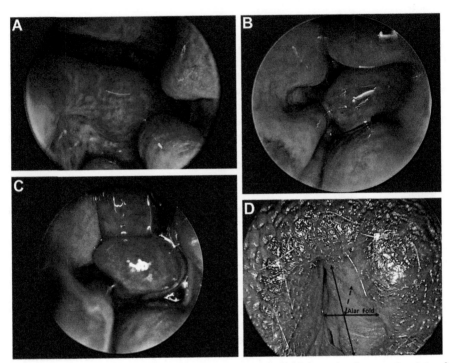

Fig. 1. Examples of crowded, hypertrophic nasal turbinates (*A*) causing increased points of mucosal contact amongst intranasal structures, rostral aberrant turbinates causing obstruction of the conducting airway (*B*) and (*C*), and close-up view of the alar fold (*D*), which is rigid and immobile in brachycephalic dogs and causes obstruction to airflow at the level of the nasal vestibule.

including neck-extended sleeping positions and the use of a toy or bone in the mouth to facilitate mouth-breathing during sleep, are most often correlated to an extremely thickened soft palate (**Fig. 3**).[23,42] Brachycephalic dogs require mechanical ventilation more often than non-brachycephalic dogs and were most frequently ventilated in 1 study for respiratory fatigue secondary to aspiration pneumonia.[50] Finally, acquired myocardial damage may be present in brachycephalic dogs—cardiac troponin-1 levels were elevated in 48% of dogs in 1 report.[51]

TRADITIONAL AND MODIFIED MULTI-LEVEL SURGERIES

To avoid secondary complications like these, it has been recommended brachycephalic dogs have corrective surgery early in life, as early as 5 months of age,[32,37,47] and diagnostics including oral and laryngoscopic examination, computed tomography (CT), and anterior and posterior rhinoscopy be performed in *all* cases to ascertain the location of all airway stenoses or abnormalities requiring correction.[7,17,32,39,52] Additionally, a modified collection of new procedures comprising multi-level upper airway surgery has received attention and merit for documented ability to achieve more promising outcomes than traditional surgeries[7,39,42] The new, modified multi-level surgery (MMS) consists of ala vestibuloplasty[44,45] (**Fig. 4**); modified folded flap palatoplasty or palatal volume reduction[18,38] (**Fig. 5**); resection or microlaryngoscopic ablation of the everted mucosa of the laryngeal ventricles; tonsillectomy, partial

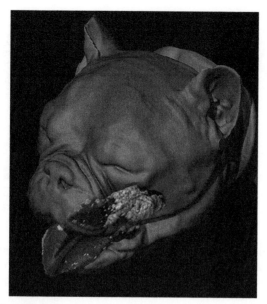

Fig. 2. Some brachycephalic breeds accumulate fat at the base of the tongue that may contribute to sleep-disordered breathing and other clinical signs of brachycephalic obstructive airway syndrome.

tonsillectomy, or tonsillotomy of the palatine tonsils; and partial laryngectomy involving cuneiformectomy in dogs with grades II or III laryngeal collapse.[7,18,39] Liu and colleagues compared traditional multi-level surgery (TMS) that combined alaplasty and staphylectomy with resection of laryngeal saccules to the modified multi-level surgery described earlier (MMS) using whole-body barometric plethysmography (WBBP), a non-invasive technique using barometric pressure oscillations to objectively measure respiratory function.[7,48] Dogs treated with traditional surgery had an 8 times greater risk of poor prognosis than dogs treated using newer MMS techniques.[7] However, even dogs treated by MMS were assessed to still have

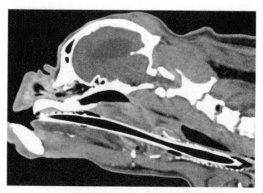

Fig. 3. Computed tomographic sagittal reconstructed image showing an extremely thickened and overlong soft palate causing both nasopharyngeal and oropharyngeal obstruction to airflow.

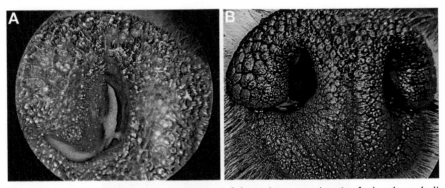

Fig. 4. Endoscopic and digital camera images of the right external naris of a brachycephalic dog before (A) and after (B) ala vestibuloplasty. Note the obstruction caused by the rigid alar fold (A).

compromised respiratory function according to BOAS indices assessed by WBBP and a validated respiratory functional grading system.[7,12,48] The authors of the study postulated that lesions untreated by even MMS such as a large tongue base, tracheal hypoplasia, and aberrant nasal conchal conformations might be to blame.[7] Regarding surgical options to address these lesions, reduction glossoplasty has only recently been proposed as a potential treatment for macroglossia in brachycephalic dogs,[53] and tissue components contributing to macroglossia and indications and prognosis for surgical treatment of macroglossia require further study before glossectomy or glossoplasty can be routinely recommended.[19,20,53] Although no known surgical treatment for tracheal hypoplasia exists, surgical treatment of abnormal conchal conformations, though not yet widely available, has been thoroughly described and intensively evaluated.[18,39,40,54]

LASER-ASSISTED TURBINECTOMY

Presently offered by only 3 surgical groups in the world, that of Dr Gerhard Oectering and colleagues at the University of Leipzig, Germany; Dr Ladlow, Liu, and colleagues at the University of Cambridge and Hamilton's Veterinary Specialists, UK; and by the author at the University of Illinois, laser-assisted turbinectomy (LATE) has shown promise as a treatment for clinical signs caused by intranasal airway obstructions due to abnormal conchae.[18,39,40,42]

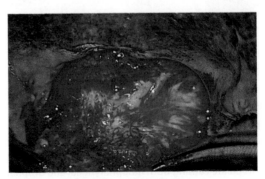

Fig. 5. Dissection plane during folded flap palatoplasty.

INTRANASAL EVALUATION

Dr Oectering and colleagues were the first to describe systematic assessment of the nasal cavity from the caudal nasal vestibule to the nasopharynx for abnormal conchal configurations.[17,32] He ascribed intranasal obstruction in brachycephalic dogs, in part, to "relative conchal hypertrophy," a situation in which the extremely foreshortened nasal cavities are too small for even appropriately sized or undersized turbinates, permitting points of mucosal contact between conchal lamellae and other mucosal structures in the nasal cavity.[17,32] Additionally, bullous conformations of conchae having sparse branches of thickened, crude lamellae[17] were found to characterize turbinates growing aberrantly into the rostral and caudal conducting airways of the nasal cavities.[17,18,32,54] The authors emphasized that thorough CT and endoscopic examination of the intranasal airways should be performed as part of surgical planning for *all* brachycephalic dogs presented for signs of BOAS and provided the following guidelines for assessment.[17,32] The surgeon should place the tip of a 1.9-mm or 2.7-mm rigid endoscope (HOPKINS II straight 0° telescope, 18 cm working length, Karl Storz Veterinary Endoscopy North America, Goleta, CA) just caudal to each right and left nasal vestibule at the opening to the nasal cavities to obtain the classic "5-fold view" of the nasal folds—the plicae recta, alaris, and basalis laterally and the dorsal and ventral septal swell bodies medially (**Fig. 6**). At this location, the authors recommended that mucosal structures be evaluated for contact between

- Individual lamellae of the ventral nasal concha (CNV), known as intraconchal contact, or lamellae of the CNV and lamellae of the middle nasal concha (CNM), known as interconchal contact,
- Either the CNV or CNM and the nasal septum,
- Lamellae of the CNV and the lateral wall,
- Lamellae of the CNV and the nasal floor,
- Either lamellae of the CNV or CNM and the plica recta,
- Lamellae of the CNV and the plica alaris,
- Lamellae of the CNV and the plica basalis.

The authors found at least 1 point of mucosal contact in 87% of the brachycephalic dogs, including 96% of the French bulldogs, in contrast to the normocephalic dogs, of

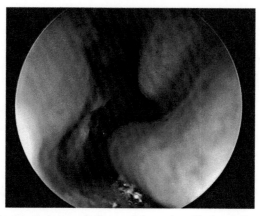

Fig. 6. Anterior rhinoscopic image at the caudal nasal vestibule of the right nasal passage showing the alar folds. Most evident are the dorsal and ventral septal swell bodies medially and the plica alaris and plica basalis laterally.

which 76% had no mucosal contact at all.[32] Pug dogs more commonly had nasal septal deviation and contact between the nasal septum and the plica recta.[32] In a subsequent landmark paper describing additional causes of intranasal airway obstruction, Oechtering and others defined turbinates as aberrant if turbinate lamellae branched into a nasal meatus and obstructed airflow.[17] Rostral aberrant turbinates (RATs) were classified as lamellae from the CNV or CNM that spread abnormally rostral to where the plica alaris first branches into the CNV, obstructing the common and middle nasal meatuses.[17] Ladlow, however, also identified RATs *caudal* to the first branch of the plica alaris that compounded obstructions already in that area due to crowded turbinates.[39] Caudal aberrant turbinates (CATs) were classified as lamellae from the CNV, CNM, or endoturbinate III that spread abnormally caudal into the nasopharyngeal meatus or nasopharynx ventral to the wing of the vomer, causing obstruction to airflow at the nasal exit.[17]

COMPUTED TOMOGRAPHIC ASSESSMENT

Auger and colleagues recently reported using CT to evaluate and compare intranasal points of mucosal contact and aberrant growth of turbinates.[47] Although 94% of all the brachycephalic dogs had points of contact among intranasal mucosal structures compared to only 9.4% of the normocephalic dogs, the authors cited several limitations. They were only able to assess the rostral one-third of the nasal cavities, as nasal contact points became "more difficult to distinguish" using CT caudally.[47] Additionally, the authors ceded that CT volume averaging artifact or overlap with nasal secretions might have accounted for the higher prevalence of what they termed "intranasal mucosal contact points" compared with endoscopic evaluation.[17,32,47] It has been this author's experience that RATs and points of mucosal contact are not easily distinguished on CT and are best observed by endoscopy, while CATs are readily visualized and graded on CT as well as anterior and posterior endoscopy (**Fig. 7**). Although all foci of intranasal obstruction are carefully qualified prior to treatment, this author makes no effort to quantify points of contact. Liu, Ladlow and others agree, reporting that consistent quantification of intranasal mucosal contact points by rhinoscopy is challenging due to the turbinates being "hypertrophied and compressed" and preventing passage of the endoscope for evaluation of the caudal one-third to half of the nasal cavity.[32,39] The same authors reported that points of mucosal contact are also difficult to quantify on CT because the conchal mucosa is too thin to be visualized on CT.[39] At the author's

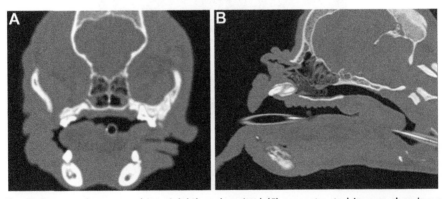

Fig. 7. Computed tomographic axial (*A*) and sagittal (*B*) reconstructed images showing a right-sided caudal aberrant turbinate contributing to obstruction of the nasopharyngeal meatus.

institution, following sedated airway examination, continuous airway CT of the head, neck, and chest is performed under general anesthesia using a 128-slice helical unit (Siemens SOMATOM Definition, Siemens Medical Solutions USA, Inc., Malvern, PA), 120 kVp, 12 mas, 0.625 mm slice thickness, a small scan field of view, 18 cm FOV, and a bone algorithm to evaluate for airway abnormalities including stenosis of the nares and nasal vestibules, prolongation and thickening of the soft palate, nasal septal deviation, CATs, nasopharyngeal cysts or polyps, tracheal hypoplasia, tracheal and bronchial collapse, aspiration pneumonia, and hiatal hernia.[49] Other aberrations not affecting the airway discernible on CT include spinal malformations and hemivertebrae, intracranial ventricular dilatation, obliteration of the frontal sinuses, stenoses of the ear canals, and changes to the tympanic bullae and middle ear.[1,17,18,32,39,49,55] The author combines CT findings with direct anterior and posterior rhinoscopy to completely characterize intranasal obstructions and to guide endoscopic-assisted surgical planning.

CANDIDACY FOR LASER-ASSISTED TURBINECTOMY

Although Oechtering and colleagues reported performing LATE as 1 essential component of MMS and never as a stand-alone procedure, MMS has been performed successfully without LATE.[7,39] A study was performed to evaluate the effectiveness of and indications for LATE in dogs affected by BOAS.[39] Dogs having abnormal intranasal structures on CT and endoscopy prior to MMS, a BOAS index of greater than 50% following MMS, and assignment of a functional grade of II or III following MMS were considered candidates for LATE.[39] Candidates for LATE had a median BOAS index of 88.8% preoperative MMS and a median BOAS index of 66.7% postoperative MMS; the BOAS index further decreased to 42.3% after the addition of LATE. Neither the presence nor severity of RATs, CATs, or septal deviation were indications for LATE. Only the cross-sectional area of the soft tissue proportion at the rostral entrance of the choanae (STC) was a predictor of candidacy for LATE.[39]

The author considers any brachycephalic dog, especially pugs, French bulldogs, and English bulldogs, to be candidates for evaluation for LATE if they have failed TMS performed by a board-certified veterinary surgeon at another institution or have persistence of clinical signs following MMS at the author's institution. Given we service a lengthy waitlist of potential candidates for LATE, to receive more timely definitive treatment, many owners travel with their dogs to the author's institution for MMS alone prior to consideration for LATE. Consequently, the author has observed that many dogs diagnosed with CATs and other abnormal conchal configurations on CT experience significant amelioration of presenting clinical signs following MMS alone. As WBBP is not widely available, the author recommends CT imaging for any dog with signs of sleep apnea or severe respiratory distress and MMS + LATE for dogs with confirmed intranasal lesions and signs of severe increases in intrathoracic negative pressure following TMS, including sucking in of the skin at the nares and thoracic inlet on inspiration; wide, bellowing excursions of the caudal ribcage on inspiration; or paradoxic respiratory motion and effort. Although no dog that has undergone MMS alone at the author's institution has subsequently required LATE, in the absence of oscillometry, pneumotachography, or plethysmography instrumentation, the author uses the validated respiratory functional grading system of Liu and Ladlow to help determine which dogs might require LATE following TMS or MMS.[48]

SYSTEMATIC EXAMINATION OF THE UPPER AIRWAYS

Concerning technical performance of LATE, Oechtering and others have published a finely detailed description of the procedure, which will not be repeated here, except to outline the steepest areas of the learning curve.[18] Firstly, a wide selection of specialized endoscopic equipment and hand tools is needed as well as training in how to use the equipment.[17,18] The author utilizes a rigid endoscopy system (Karl Storz Veterinary Endoscopy North America, Goleta, CA), beginning with the sedated laryngoscopic examination. A direct visual oral examination as well as laryngoscopic examination (HOPKINS II, 0°, 18 cm enlarged view telescope, Karl Storz Veterinary Endoscopy North America, Goleta, CA) is performed. The oropharyngeal area is assessed for macroglossia, everted mucosa of the laryngeal saccules (grade I laryngeal collapse), elongation of the soft palate beyond the tip of the epiglottis or caudal aspect of the palatine tonsils, enlargement and eversion of the palatine tonsils, structural or mucosal laryngeal lesions, and higher grades of laryngeal collapse. Every patient undergoes further examination by the addition of doxapram HCl (Dopram-V; Fort Dodge Laboratories, Fort Dodge, IA,USA; 1.1 mg kg) 0.55 to 1.1 mg/kg IV to further assess laryngeal function.[56,57] For dogs initially exhibiting criteria of grades II or III laryngeal collapse or paradoxic motion of the corniculate or cuneiform processes of the arytenoid cartilages, the author always gives a full 1.1 mg/kg IV dose of doxapram. It has been the author's experience that many dogs with paradoxic motion or concern for higher grades of laryngeal collapse on initial examination will reverse course on full dosing with doxapram, without adverse effects on heart rate or blood pressure,[57] converting from paradoxic to normal laryngeal function or from higher grades of laryngeal collapse to grade I laryngeal collapse. (Video 2) Judgment of laryngeal function is therefore reserved until observation following 1.1 mg/kg doxapram administration has been performed.[56,57]

Patients are then intubated and transported for CT examination. Continuous airway CT of the head, neck, and chest is performed, and images are assessed for abnormalities as described earlier. Most patients presented to the author's clinic for LATE have undergone TMS, but not MMS, and while MMS + LATE are generally performed in 1 session, LATE is performed prior to all other procedures. Dogs are placed in sternal recumbency with the maxilla slung by a cord that is itself slung over a custom frame fixed to the surgical table (Fig. 8). For French and English bulldogs and brachycephalic dogs of similar size, a 30°, HOPKINS II forward-oblique, 18-cm, 2.7-mm diameter telescope (Karl Storz Veterinary Endoscopy North America, Goleta, CA) is passed through each nasal vestibule to the entrance of the right and left nasal passages to obtain the "5-fold view;" a 1.9-mm telescope might be required for Boston terriers, pugs, other smaller breeds of dog, and cats. The origin of any RAT is noted, as is the severity of intranasal contact of mucosal structures. Photographs are taken to document the presence and severity of airway obstruction. A pot of dilute iodine solution and separate pot of sterile saline are sequentially useful for frequent cleansing of the telescope lens of blood or other fluids, followed by wiping with gauze. Application of an antifogging solution to the lens also provides more consistent clarity (Dr Clear AntiFog Set, Karl Storz Veterinary Endoscopy North America, Goleta, CA). Flushing of the nasal cavities with saline is avoided during rhinoscopy for LATE to avoid incitation of mucosal edema, other changes to mucosal structures, obscuring of the telescope lens with fluid, and increased risk for aspiration.[18] To most accurately evaluate and treat obstructive nasal conchal configurations all the way through the nasopharyngeal meatus to the nasopharynx, an alpha agonist such as oxymetazoline 0.05% 0.2 to 0.4 mL is sprayed into each nasal cavity to induce nasal turbinate decongestion by vasoconstriction.[54] Vasoconstriction and decongestion confer key advantages to the endoscopist; first, to shrink the turbinate tissues, allowing for easier navigation through the nasal passages, and second, to limit significant hemorrhage from constricted vessels (Fig. 9)[54,58,59] While waiting for the nasal decongestant to take effect

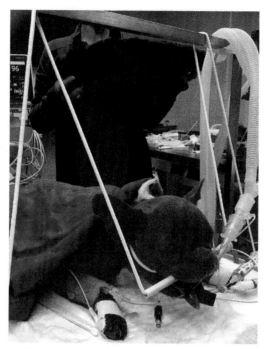

Fig. 8. Dogs are placed in sternal recumbency with the maxilla slung by a cord that is itself slung over a custom frame fixed to the surgical table.

over approximately 5 minutes, the lumens of each nasopharyngeal meatus, the choanae, and nasopharynx are examined by posterior rhinoscopy and a 120°, HOPKINS II rigid 18-cm, 4-mm diameter retrograde telescope (Karl Storz Veterinary Endoscopy North America, Goleta, CA). It is expected and has been the author's experience that CATs detected on CT within the nasopharyngeal meatus or extending to the nasopharynx should be able to be visualized by endoscopy in all cases.[17]

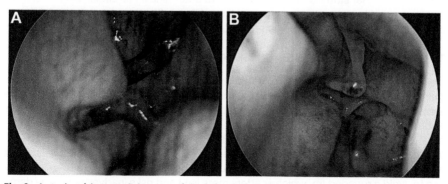

Fig. 9. Anterior rhinoscopic images of the left nasal passage showing crowded, hypertrophic turbinates causing increased points of mucosal contact before (A) and after (B) administration of 0.2 to 0.4 mL oxymetazoline 0.05% sprayed intranasally. Vasoconstrictive and decongestant effects result in turbinate lamellae that are paler and shrunken compared to pre-administration.

PERFORMING LASER-ASSISTED TURBINECTOMY

LATE is begun with either nasal cavity; the author generally starts with the most affected nasal cavity based on CT and endoscopic evaluation. Oechtering and colleagues described 3 parts to the original LATE procedure for dogs with intranasal lesions severely affected by BOAS: turbinectomy of the CNV for relative hypertrophy of the CNV causing multiple points of mucosal contact and/or RATs originating from the CNV, resection of the CNM for RATs originating from the CNM, and turbinectomy of CATs originating from the CNV, CNM, or EIII.[18] Oechtering and others also described a CAT-specific procedure, termed "CAT LATE," for dogs with minimally obstructive intranasal conchae and few, if any, points of mucosal contact, but with CATs originating from the CNM or EIII causing obstruction at the nasal exit.[54] Given the physiologic benefit that might result from preserving the thermoregulatory function of the CNV, CAT LATE was designed to spare the CNV in cases where CATs originate from the CNM or EIII.[18,54] However, in cases were RATs or CATs do arise from the CNV, or in cases where the CNV lamellae are hypertrophic and contribute to intranasal obstruction, the CNV must undergo turbinectomy.[18,54]

Vilaplana Grosso and colleagues described a 5-point grading scheme of CATs based on CT.[60] Dogs were given a classification grade of "0" if no turbinates were identified in the ventral nasal meatus, "1" if turbinates were visible in the ventral nasal meatus rostral to the point of branching of the basal lamina of the ethmoid bone with the perpendicular lamina of the palatine bone at the entrance to the nasopharyngeal meatus, "2" if turbinates were noted in the nasopharyngeal meatus without extension through the choanae to the nasopharynx, "3" if turbinates were visible in the choanae at the caudal border of the vomer but not extending past the end of the nasal septum, and "4" if turbinates extended past the choanae and end of the nasal septum into the nasopharynx.[60] The authors of this study only evaluated English bulldogs but found 100% of the dogs to have CATs as defined earlier, with 70% having grade 2 CATs, but no clinical signs of respiratory disease.[60] Ladlow and others also found CATs in 100% of 57 pugs and French and English bulldogs treated for LATE, and, using the Vilaplana Grosso classification system, found no correlation between CAT classification and candidacy for LATE[39] However, in their study of 24 pugs and 1 English bulldog, Oechtering and others reported that all CATs treated by CAT LATE would have fallen into grades 3 and 4 if classified according to the Vilaplana Grosso scheme.[54] Further study is therefore needed to determine if this classification scheme can be applied to all brachycephalic breeds and if classification may be a useful determinant of which dogs might benefit from LATE or CAT LATE.[39,54,60]

TURBINECTOMY OF THE VENTRAL NASAL CONCHA

Oechtering reported that ablation of the CNV should begin immediately rostral to the point at which the plica alaris first branches into the CNV and where RATs had been identified.[18] However, Ladlow and colleagues also found RATs caudal to this branch to be exacerbating the obstruction already present due to relative hypertrophy of turbinates.[39] Regardless, to perform LATE, a diode laser (980-nm wavelength and 10–30-W total power) with 400-um fiber is used at a setting of 3 to 4 W in continuous wave mode.[18,39,54] The laser fiber should be cut sharply with a diamond cutter prior to use to avoid a rounded tip, which scatters more light and risks inadvertent tissue damage.[18] It is recommended to use the laser in both contact and non-contact modes during LATE to accomplish a variety of laser light-tissue interactions.[18] Because 980-nm wavelength light penetrates intact mucosa and is absorbed by deeper layers of tissue, 1 dissection technique involves using the laser in near-contact mode with a stand-off of approximately 0.5 to 2 mm. This technique results in more coagulation than cutting and is useful for achieving hemostasis of deep vessels as well as volume reduction or sculpting of turbinates in contact with other mucosal structures (Video 3).[18] Alternatively, using the laser in contact mode creates a more focused, power dense beam that forms a thin carbonized layer of tissue (Video 4). Because carbonized tissue has a higher absorption coefficient for diode laser light, subsequent withdrawal of the laser tip from contact turbinate mucosa permits further absorption of laser light and generation of sufficient energy to cut tissue, even in non-contact mode.[18] Such a "mixed mode" of coagulation and cutting permits dissection of tissue after blood vessels have been coagulated, a wise approach to the highly vascularized tissues of the nasal conchae.[18]

During LATE, the efficiency of turbinate resection and volume reduction is dictated by several factors—the tiny space of the brachycephalic nasal cavity; use of the endoscope, the lens of which constrains the field of view and frequently requires cleaning; the generation of hemorrhage and smoke on lasing; and the skill of the endoscopist in mitigating these factors. As nasal flushing through the endoscope sheath may compromise the appearance of the nasal tissue and lead to local edema and systemic complications, hemorrhage and smoke should be primarily controlled by suction.[18] Passing a soft tipped suction catheter such as a red rubber catheter through the contralateral naris to position the open tip past the nasal septum may help to remove smoke and hemorrhage generated on incision of turbinate tissue from the operated nasal passage through the common nasopharynx.[18] Alternatively, and specifically for hemorrhage, the author has found placing a red rubber catheter ventrally in the ipsilateral nasal cavity and rotating the side hole helpto clear the field of blood and smoke (Video 5). Additionally, maintaining an ipsilaterally placed ventral catheter helps to hold open the nasal vestibule and provides a guide for ready passage of the scope directly to the ventral nasal meatus.

Bleeding from the CNV is most likely to be profuse at its caudal aspect where the sphenopalatine artery enters.[18] Use of the laser in non-contact mode to blanch the tissue and induce a coagulum before transection is helpful. If bleeding still occurs, suctioning with the side hole of the red rubber catheter while lasing can be helpful to isolate and ablate the source of hemorrhage. Alternatively, as Oechtering recommends, an open-ended suction pipe can be used on the bleeding tissue immediately adjacent to the point of hemorrhage to manipulate the tissue and bring it in contact with the laser fiber.[18]

As pieces of the CNV or other conchal tissue are transected, they can be grasped and removed with Heermann ear forceps,[18] microalligator forceps, or microcutting cup forceps. The author prefers curved microalligator forceps for their versatility and ease of applicability at multiple angles (Video 6). Hemostasis may be achieved using all the afore-mentioned mechanisms throughout the LATE procedure as required.

Oechtering describes use of a rigid suction pipe not only for evacuation of fluids such as blood, nasal secretions, or residual oxymetazoline or other alpha agonist, but also as a means by which to "grasp" the tissue to be resected and position it in line for transection.[18] Because Oechtering reports operating the endoscope through the sheath with the laser fiber passed through the working channel, the scope and laser must work in parallel and cannot be brought in alignment with the tissue; rather the tissue must be brought into alignment with the scope, sheath, and laser.[18] The suction pipe provides a convenient means by which to accomplish this, offering gentle, adhesive grasping of the tissue while also delineating attachments for dissection and suctioning smoke, blood, and other byproducts of laser dissection (Video 7).[18] Additionally, constraining the scope and laser fiber within the endoscope sheath consolidates instrumentation and may simplify movements. However, the author has found that reliance on the familiar interaction of instruments that are *triangulated*, even within the very small space of the nasal cavity, is helpful for any surgeon just beginning to become familiar with intranasal anatomy, airway trajectories, the relative position of normal and abnormal intranasal structures, and the responses of nasal tissues to diode laser light and endoscopic-assisted manipulation. Limited triangulation *is possible* even through a stenotic naris and within the small brachycephalic nasal cavity when the endoscope is passed *without* a sheath and the laser is threaded through a handpiece with angled tip. Curved microalligator forceps may be exchanged for the laser handpiece for removal of laser-resected turbinate tissue.

Conchae, especially the CNV, have important physiologic functions, including the warming, moistening, and filtering of air. Turbinates also function in odor discrimination, endurance, social behavior, and most importantly, thermoregulation.[1,40] In a panting dog, blood is cooled as it traverses the arteriovenous anastomoses of the CNV and flows into the internal rete of the cavernous sinus, lowering the temperature of blood in the internal carotid artery by counter flow heat exchange.[61] The importance of thermoregulation is underscored by Ladlow's observation that increased soft tissue proportion at the rostral entrance to the choanae, the site of the lateral nasal gland, was the only significant predictor of candidacy for LATE.[39] The authors speculated that enlargement of the lateral nasal gland, seen on CT as an increase in soft tissue proportion, was a compensatory response to poor thermoregulation associated with intranasal obstruction.[39] While removal of the CNV disrupts evaporative heat exchange and thermoregulation, a hypertrophic or aberrantly growing CNV must yet be removed in many brachycephalic dogs to critically improve airflow.[54] Interestingly, dogs that underwent CNV ablation experienced hypertrophy of the *CNM* by the time of the 6 month reevaluation in 1 study, but only if the CNM had remained untouched during LATE.[40] A hypertrophic CNM may increase the surface area available following LATE for evaporative cooling and thermoregulation, but may also contribute to recurrence of intranasal obstruction.[40,54] Regrowth of healthy, non-obstructive, functional turbinates from conchal remnants of an ablated CNV would be desirable but is unlikely according to current research.[18,40] As a result, radical resection of turbinates from nasal conchae, especially the CNV and CNM, is not recommended.[40]

TURBINECTOMY OF ROSTRAL ABERRANT TURBINATES DERIVING FROM THE MIDDLE NASAL CONCHA

RATs originating from the CNV will have been removed by ablation of the CNV for treatment of relative hypertrophy and increased points of mucosal contact. RATs originating from the CNM, however, may be unstable and settle ventrally into the ventral nasal meatus where they should be removed.[18] Laser dissection for removal of the CNM should begin where the CNM emerges laterally, close to the sphenoid sinus.[18,40]

TURBINECTOMY OF CAUDAL ABERRANT TURBINATES

It has been stated that CATs should be removed to clear the nasopharyngeal meatus and nasopharynx of obstructing turbinate tissue to decrease intranasal resistance[17,18,54] The author has removed CATs by anterior rhinoscopy using a 30°, HOPKINS II forward-oblique, 18-cm, 1.9-mm or 2.7-mm diameter telescope (Karl Storz Veterinary Endoscopy North America, Goleta, CA). CATs derived from the CNV will also already have been removed by this stage of the LATE procedure.[18,54] CATs derived from the CNM or EIII, however, hang into the nasopharyngeal meatus and can be laser-resected from either turbinate by dissecting with great care where the

CAT curves into the nasopharyngeal meatus (see **Fig. 7**). Once dissected, CATs can be removed by grasping with hand instruments as described earlier.[18,54] The author prefers curved microalligator forceps which can be more readily manipulated than straight grasping forceps to accommodate the plane of dissection this far caudally in the nose.

The LATE procedure may subsequently be considered complete if the ventral conducting airway from the nasal vestibule to the nasopharyngeal meatus and nasopharynx is free of obstructing hypertrophic or aberrant turbinates, and the arch-shaped rostral opening to the nasopharyngeal meatus is clear (Video 8).[18,54] The author has found that hypertrophic and aberrant turbinate tissue may settle into the conducting airways during dissection but become hidden by blood clots adherent to the lateral wall of the nasal cavity, and thorough flushing of the area with sterile saline followed by suction and gentle inspection by probing the lateral walls of the nasal passages should be performed prior to completion of the procedure.

CAT-specific LATE has also been described in detail by Oechtering and colleagues[54] Performing CAT LATE and not a full LATE procedure spares the CNV in operated dogs, which, as discussed, features prominently in preserving thermoregulatory processes.[18] The author's caseload is dominated by French bulldogs, whose pathology typically consists of relative hypertrophy of CNV turbinates causing intranasal obstruction, RATs originating from the CNV, and CATs originating from the CNV, or less often the CNM.[17,18,54] These pathologies are indications for a full LATE procedure and not CAT LATE.[54] It has been reported that pugs, unlike French bulldogs, commonly have CATs without other significant nasal pathology, and so CAT LATE appears to be most applicable to this breed at this time.[54]

INTRAOPERATIVE AND POSTOPERATIVE COMPLICATIONS
Intraoperative Complications

Complications related to LATE alone appear to be relatively minor compared to complications reported more broadly for brachycephalic patients undergoing TMS or MMS without LATE.[2,4–7,22–24] Because LATE is never performed as a solitary procedure, but only as part of MMS at all institutions where it is presently offered as treatment,[18,39] it is not possible to discern what, if any, complications can be solely ascribed to LATE. However, 1 complication experienced variably by the author, minor hemorrhage, is to be expected during operation of vascular structures and is generally abated by flushing with cold saline, additional lasing, or tamponade with a cotton swab and tincture of time. Oechtering and colleagues reported bleeding from the sphenopalatine artery sufficient to impair visualization and require flushing with cold saline or tamponade with a gauze pack in 51/158 (32.3%) pugs, French bulldogs, and English bulldogs; bleeding was not more common in any 1 breed.[18] In another report, bleeding in 1 dog was sufficient to impair visualization and required abortion of the procedure, which was completed successfully 1 week later.[54] Other complications include unintentional lasing of nearby structures including the floor of the nasal cavity or nasopharynx or of the nasal septum.[18,54] Aberrant applications of laser light presumably led to adhesion formation in some dogs noted on second-look endoscopy 6 months postoperatively.[18] These were most common between the rostral plica recta and dorsal swell body and also reported between the CNM and nasal septum (**Fig. 10**).[18] Adhesions were readily broken down by blunt detachment without clinical consequence.[18,54]

Lastly, intraoperative death occurred in 0.8% of the dogs in 1 report due to anesthetic complications in 2 cases.[18]

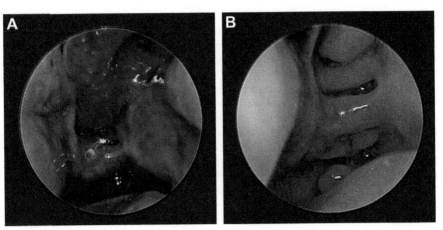

Fig. 10. Anterior rhinoscopic images of the left nasal passage showing adhesion between the plica alaris and nasal septum, presumably due to aberrant application of diode laser light. After administration of oxymetazoline (*B*), the adhesion was amenable to treatment by incision and sculpting of the nasal mucosa by laser dissection using contact and non-contact modes, respectively.

Postoperative Complications

Reported postoperative complications include self-limiting reverse sneezing in 60% of dogs, a finding not previously reported following TMS or MMS for treatment of BOAS.[39] The authors attributed this finding to increased sniffing in the postoperative period combined with a more rapid flow of air through a narrow and collapsible nasopharynx, causing vibration of soft tissues.[39] Reverse sneezing has been reported to be a physiologic cleaning procedure of the nasopharyngeal airway and may result from nasal mucosal irritation and nasal discharge induced by LATE.[62]

Mild nasal discharge and scabbing were noted in 150/158 (nearly 85%) dogs reported by Oechtering and colleagues[18] As ala vestibuloplasty can also result in mild nasal discharge and scabbing, and as LATE is performed as part of MMS that includes ala vestibuloplasty, it cannot be ascertained whether LATE alone causes nasal discharge. However, the author prefers to keep LATE patients hospitalized for 4 to 5 days following MMS + LATE as most owners and dogs travel from a distance. During the hospitalization period, the author has observed that nasal discharge associated with MMS + LATE is slightly more significant in volume and opacity than nasal discharge associated with ala vestibuloplasty. The latter is often clear, serosanguinous discharge causing mild crusting along the axial cut edges of the alar wing and alar fold. The author has attributed the slightly increased volume and opacity of nasal discharge in patients having undergone MMS + LATE to sloughing of nasal mucosa associated with laser-induced carbonization of tissue as well as tissue turnover that occurs during the mucosalization process. LATE-associated nasal discharge generally does not cause respiratory issues, is readily monitored and cleansed by owners following a minor tutorial on postoperative care, and generally resolves over a 4 to 6 week postoperative period.

The author has noted complications in 2 dogs attributed to stimulation of the vagal reflex during the operation. In both cases, the dogs showed a rapidly progressive bradycardia during LATE that progressed to cardiac arrest. Each incident was caught early and responded well to atropine administration and brief application of chest compressions with continued mechanical ventilation. This complication was also reported by Liu and colleagues and is likely due to vagal hypersensitivity associated with prolonged breathing against both fixed and dynamic upper airway obstructions, causing pathologic increases in negative airway and intrathoracic pressures, profound inspiratory effort, and airway inflammation[39] In both of the author's cases, the MMS + LATE procedure was aborted, the dogs returned home, and were re-presented by their owners for completion of the MMS + LATE procedure after several months. Temporary transvenous pacemakers were implanted into both patients before the second procedure, and both second procedures continued uneventfully to completion with very satisfactory results.

Postoperative temporary tracheostomy tube placement has been rarely required following LATE. Of 203 dogs reported to have undergone LATE or CAT LATE, only 2 (1.0%) pug dogs with grade 3 laryngeal collapse required temporary tracheostomy,[18,39,54] compared to 1.6% to 6% of dogs that had undergone TMS in various reports.[34,36,63–65] In the author's experience, only 1 French bulldog required temporary tracheostomy following MMS + LATE. In all 3 dogs, the tracheostomy tube was able to be removed after 48 hours without complication.[39] No dogs required permanent tracheostomy.

Two dogs (0.8%) died in the early recovery period according to 1 report.[18] Postoperative death was ascribed to laryngeal obstruction due to excitement, a complication that has been reported following TMS for treatment of BOAS and cannot be solely attributed to performance of LATE.[18,22,23] At the time of writing, no dogs have died in the postoperative period following MMS + LATE at the author's institution. However, since excitement is a risk for any hospitalized brachycephalic dog,[22,23] the author prefers to begin all BOAS patients on a sedation protocol preoperatively at the time of admission including trazodone 3 to 5 mg/kg PO q8-12h. Following surgery, acepromazine 0.005 to 0.01 mg/kg is administered IV q4-6 PRN, and is preferred over dexmedetomidine, as the latter may cause more relaxation of pharyngeal musculature and inhibition of the swallowing reflex.[66]

PROGNOSIS

At 6 months postoperative, ~84% of the dogs in the Oechtering report had patent nasal airways, but ~16% of the dogs had conchal regrowth sufficient to result in intranasal airway obstruction and require re-operation of 1 or both nasal passages.[18] Following MMS + LATE performed by Ladlow and others, the BOAS index remained greater than 50% in 4/20 (20%) dogs; all 4 of these dogs had some degree of laryngeal collapse.[39] Of 18 owners that returned completed postoperative questionnaires, 17 owners reported their dog was able to walk or play longer after LATE, including 3 of 4 dogs that were given a suboptimal score on the BOAS index post-LATE.[39] Sleep disturbances resolved following LATE in all dogs that had sleep-disordered breathing. All 18 owners were satisfied or very satisfied with their dogs' outcomes.[39] In another study, results of a quality-of-life questionnaire indicated most dogs with severe brachycephaly improved markedly after MMS + LATE.[42] Breathing sounds and sleep disturbances decreased substantially, and there was a marked reduction in life-threatening events such as collapse and choking fits.[42]

Theories as to why brachycephalic dogs develop aberrant turbinates or hypertrophic conchae to the point of intranasal obstruction may also help to explain conchal regrowth after MMS + LATE. While brachycephaly is characterized by arrest of craniofacial development in the postnatal period, nasal conchae grow predominantly after birth, and it is suspected that conchae have potential for growth throughout a pet's life and can adapt patterns of growth due to airway input or stimuli.[18,32,40] Nasal conchae should terminate growth in a normal dog before surfaces from adjacent mucosal structures come into contact.[17,40] As conchal cells appear to respond to airflow, lack of airflow, or changes in airflow and associated alterations in airway pressures and shear stresses,[32] failure of turbinate growth to terminate appropriately in brachycephalic dogs likely results from early reduced airflow and diminished shear stresses related to stenosis of the nares and nasal vestibular stenosis.[17] It is possible that the physical stresses needed to signal turbinate growth termination may not occur in these obstructed nasal passages until some degree of mucosal contact occurs.[40]

Turbinates likely develop aberrantly into RATs and CATs because the foreshortened nose offers little space in which to grow normally, forcing conchae to grow in aberrant paths and patterns.[32,44] Conchae that are grossly abnormally configured are also histologically abnormal. Aberrant turbinate lamellae or those contributing to mucosal contact and intranasal obstruction have thicker underlying bone and thickened mucosa with enlarged vessels and fewer branches compared to turbinates of normocephalic dogs.[32,40]

Oechtering proposed 2 theories of conchal regrowth after evaluating 80 pugs and French bulldogs 6 months following LATE.[40] One theory is of compensatory hypertrophy, where turbinates grow to fill open space in an effort to restore laminar airflow, avoid turbulent airflow, and mitigate dryness and crusting.[39,40] The most significant regrowth was reported in dogs with the most mucosal contact, and likely the most turbinate tissue resected.[40] Hypertrophy of the intact CNM that occurred in some dogs following ablation of the CNV may be an example of compensatory hypertrophy with the CNM assuming some of the physiologic function of the CNV.[18,40] Compensatory hypertrophy has been noted in pug dogs and people with septal deviations on the concave side, where the deviation results in more open space and potential for airflow turbulence.[32,39,40] True regeneration of turbinates, as opposed to hypertrophy of existing turbinates, may occur, but remnants of resected turbinates did not appear to be able to form completely new conchal lamellae in dogs that were revaluated.[40] Additional gross and histologic study with longer term follow-up is required to determine the pathoetiology and mechanisms of conchal regrowth following LATE for treatment of BOAS. Some mild, non-obstructive conchal regrowth would be ideal to assist in thermoregulation and other physiologic functions of the nasal conchae.[18] However, to avoid regrowth to the point of obstruction, it is prudent during LATE to remove only those conchal lamellae causing obstruction of the ventral conducting airway to preserve conchal function and prevent compensatory responses to alterations in airflow.[17,32,40,54]

CLINICS CARE POINTS

- Recent studies have ascertained that primary components of BOAS also include nasal vestibular stenosis due to a rigid, immobile alar fold; crowded, hypertrophic nasal turbinates causing increased points of mucosal contact amongst intranasal structures; and aberrant rostral and caudal nasopharyngeal turbinates causing obstruction of the conducting intranasal and nasopharyngeal airways, and these additional components should be considered during treatment planning.

- All brachycephalic dogs with moderate to severe respiratory symptoms of upper airway obstruction, especially signs of sleep-disordered breathing, should undergo sedated airway examination with doxapram 0.55 to 1.1 mg/kg IV; airway CT including the head, neck, and chest; and anterior and posterior rhinoscopy to evaluate for all primary and secondary components of BOAS known to result in upper airway obstruction

- Laser-assisted turbinectomy should be considered for any brachycephalic dog with confirmed intranasal abnormalities on CT and endoscopy and/or failure to respond to modified multi-level upper airway surgery including ala vestibuloplasty; modified folded flap palatoplasty or palatal volume reduction; resection or microlaryngoscopic ablation of the everted mucosa of the laryngeal ventricles; tonsillectomy, partial tonsillectomy, or tonsillotomy of the palatine tonsils; and partial laryngectomy involving cuneiformectomy in dogs with grades II or III laryngeal collapse.
- In these dogs, in the absence of advanced equipment for oscillometry, pneumotachography, or plethysmography, the respiratory functional grading scheme advanced by Ladlow and colleagues is a physical examination-based assessment shown to be a useful indicator for candidacy for LATE.

DISCLOSURE

The author has no commercial or financial conflicts of interest.

SUPPLEMENTARY DATA

Supplementary data related to this article can be found online at. https://doi.org/10.1016/j.cvsm.2024.02.002

REFERENCES

1. Selba MC, GU Oechtering, Heng HG, et al. The impact of selection for facial reduction in dogs: Geometric morphometric analysis of canine cranial shape. Anat Rec 2020;303:330–46.
2. Hendricks JC. Brachycephalic airway syndrome. Vet Clin North Am Small Anim Pract 1992;22(5):1145–53.
3. Asher L, Diesel G, Summers JF. Inherited defects in pedigree dogs. Part 1: Disorders related to breed standards. Vet J 2009;182:402–11.
4. Bernaerts F, Talavera T, Leemans J. Description of original endoscopic findings and respiratory functional assessment using barometric whole-body plethysmography in dogs suffering from brachycephalic airway obstruction syndrome. Vet J 2010;183:95–102.
5. Packer RAM, Hendricks A, Tivers MS, et al. Impact of facial conformation on canine health: brachycephalic obstructive airway syndrome. PLoS One 2015. https://doi.org/10.1371/journal.pone.0137496.
6. Dupre G, Heidenreich D. Brachycephalic syndrome. Vet Clin North Am Small Anim Pract 2016;46:691–707.
7. Liu N-C, GU Oechtering, Adams VJ, et al. Outcomes and prognostic factors of surgical treatments for brachycephalic obstructive airway syndrome in 3 breeds. Vet Surg 2017;46:271–80.
8. Koch D, Wiestner T, Balli A, et al. Proposal for a new radiological index to determine skull conformation in the dog. Schweiz Arch Tierheilkd 2012;154(5):217–20.
9. Evans HE, de Lahunta A. The skeleton. In: Evans HE, de Lahunta A, editors. Miller's anatomy of the dog. 4th edition. St Louis: Elsevier Saunders; 2013. p. 80–157.
10. Breed Registration Statistics. 2020. Available at: https://www.thekennelclub.org.uk/registration/breed-registration-statistics/. [Accessed 5 October 2021].
11. Meola SD. Brachycephalic airway syndrome. Top Companion Anim Med 2013;28:91–6.

12. Liu N-C, Sargan DR, Adams VJ, et al. Characterization of brachycephalic obstructive airway syndrome in French bulldogs using whole-body barometric plethysmography. PLoS One 2015. https://doi.org/10.1371/journal.pone.0130741.

13. AKC Most Popular Breeds. 2022. Available at: https://www.akc.org/most-popular-breeds/. [Accessed 6 November 2023].

14. Gleason HE, Phillips H, McCoy AM. Influence of feline brachycephaly on respiratory, gastrointestinal, sleep, and activity abnormalities. Vet Surg 2023;52(3):435–45.

15. Gleason HE, Phillips H, Fries R, et al. Ala vestibuloplasty improves cardiopulmonary and activity-related parameters in brachycephalic cats. Vet Surg 2023;52(4):575–86.

16. CFA Most Popular Breeds. 2019. Available at: https://cfa.org/cfa-news-releases/top-breeds-2019/. [Accessed 6 November 2023].

17. GU Oechtering, Pohl S, Schlueter C, et al. A novel approach to brachycephalic syndrome. 1. Evaluation of anatomical intranasal airway obstruction. Vet Surg 2016;45:165–72.

18. GU Oechtering, Pohl S, Schlueter C, et al. A novel approach to brachycephalic syndrome. 2. Laser-assisted turbinectomy (LATE). Vet Surg 2016;45:173–81.

19. Jones BA, Stanley BJ, Nelson NC. The impact of tongue dimension on air volume in brachycephalic dogs. Vet Surg 2020;49(3):512–20.

20. Song A, Phillips H, Oliveira CR, et al. CT volumetric analysis permits comparison of tongue size and tongue fat in different canine brachycephalic and mesaticephalic breeds. Vet Radiol Ultrasound 2023;1–10.

21. Ginn JA, Kumar MSA, McKiernan BC, et al. Nasopharyngeal turbinates in brachycephalic dogs and cats. J Am Anim Hosp Assoc 2008;44:243–9.

22. Fasanella FJ, Shivley JM, Wardlaw JL, et al. Brachycephalic airway obstructive syndrome in dogs: 90 cases (1991–2008). J Am Vet Med Assoc 2010;237:1048–51.

23. Roedler FS, Pohl S, GU Oechtering. How does severe brachycephaly affect dog's lives? Results of a structured preoperative owner questionnaire. Vet J 2013;198:606–10.

24. Pratschke K. Current thinking about brachycephalic syndrome: more than just airways. Comput Animat 2014;19:70–8.

25. Hoareau GL, Jourdan G, Mellema M, et al. Evaluation of arterial blood gases and arterial Blood pressures in brachycephalic dogs. J Vet Intern Med 2012;26:897–904.

26. Harvey CE. Upper airway obstruction surgery. 2. Soft palate resection in brachycephalic dogs. J Am Anim Hosp Assoc 1982;18:538–44.

27. Aron DN, Crowe DT. Upper airway obstruction. General principles and selected conditions in the dog and cat. Vet Clin North Am Small Anim Pract 1985;15:891–7.

28. Harvey CE. Surgical correction of stenotic nares in a cat. J Am Anim Hosp Assoc 1986;22:31.

29. Hobson HP. Brachycephalic syndrome. Semin Vet Med Surg Small Anim 1995;10(2):109114.

30. Brdecka DJ, Rawlings CA, Perry AC, et al. Use of an electrothermal, feedback controlled, bipolar sealing device for resection of the elongated portion of the soft palate in dogs with obstructive upper airway disease. J Am Vet Med Assoc 2008;233(8):1265–9.

31. Trappler M, Moore K. Canine brachycephalic airway syndrome: pathophysiology, diagnosis, and nonsurgical management. Compend Contin Educ Vet 2011;33(5): E1–4, quizE5.

32. Schuenemann R, GU R Oechtering. Inside the brachycephalic nose: Intranasal mucosal contact points. J Am Anim Hosp Assoc 2014;50:149–58.

33. Harvey C, Venker-von Haagan A. Surgical management of pharyngeal and laryngeal airway obstruction in the dog. Vet Clin North Am Small Anim Pract 1975;5: 515–35.

34. Poncet CM, Dupre GP, Freiche VG, et al. Long-term results of upper respiratory syndrome surgery and gastrointestinal tract medical treatment in 51 brachycephalic dogs. J Small Anim Pract 2006;47(3):137–42.

35. Torrez CV, Hunt GB. Results of surgical correction of abnormalities associated with brachycephalic airway obstruction syndrome in dogs in Australia. J Small Anim Pract 2006;47(3):150–4.

36. Riecks TW, Birchard SJ, Stephens JA. Surgical correction of brachycephalic syndrome in dogs: 62 cases (1991-2004). J Am Vet Med Assoc 2007;230(9):1324–8.

37. Oshita R, Katayose S, Kanai E, et al. Assessment of nasal structure using CT imaging of brachycephalic dog breeds. Animals 2022;12:1636–45.

38. Findji L, Dupre G. Folded flap palatoplasty for treatment of elongated soft palates in 55 dogs. Vet Med Austria 2008;95:56–63.

39. Liu N-C, Genain M-A, Klmar L, et al. Objective effectiveness of and indications for laser-assisted turbinectomy in brachycephalic obstructive airway syndrome. Vet Surg 2019;48:79–87.

40. Schuenemann R, GU Oechtering. Inside the brachycephalic nose: conchal regrowth and mucosal contact points after laser-assisted turbinectomy. J Am Anim Hosp Assoc 2014;50:237–46.

41. Lippert JP, Reinhold P, Smith HJ, et al. Geometry and function of the dog nose: how does function change when form of the nose is changed? Pneumologie 2010;64(7):452–3.

42. Pohl S, Roedler FS, GU Oechtering. How does multilevel upper airway surgery influence the lives of dogs with severe brachycephaly? Results of a structured pre- and postoperative owner questionnaire. Vet J 2016;210:39–45.

43. Hostnik ET, Scansen BA, Zielinski R, et al. Quantification of nasal airflow resistance in English bulldogs using computed tomography and computational fluid dynamics. Vet Radiol Ultrasound 2017;58(5):542–51.

44. GU Oechtering. Brachycephalic syndrome- new information on an old congenital disease. Vet Focus 2010;20(2):2–9.

45. Oechtering G, Scheunemann R. Brachycephalics: trapped in man-made misery? Turbinate Ablation in BAOS. Cambridge, UK: Proceedings of association of veterinary soft tissue surgeons autumn scientific meetings; 2010. p. 28–32.

46. Liu NC, Troconis EL, Kalmar L, et al. Conformational risk factors of brachycephalic obstructive airway syndrome (BOAS) in pugs, French bulldogs, and bulldogs. PLoS One 2017;12(8):e0181928.

47. Auger M, Alexander K, Beauchamp G, et al. Use of CT to evaluate and compare intranasal features in brachycephalic and normal dogs. J Small Anim Pract 2016; 57:529–36.

48. Riggs J, Liu N-C, Sutton DR, et al. Validation of exercise testing and laryngeal auscultation for grading brachycephalic obstructive airway syndrome in pugs, French bulldogs, and English bulldogs by using whole-body barometric plethysmography. Vet Surg 2019;48:488–96.

49. De Carhalvo IC, dos Santos Filho M, Hainfellner DC, et al. Brachycephalic syndrome in dogs- Endoscopic findings in the airways. Acta Sci Vet 2022;50: 1869–80.

50. Hoareau GL, Mellema MS, Silverstein DC. Indication, management, and outcome of brachycephalic dogs requiring mechanical ventilation. J Vet Emerg Crit Care 2011;21:226–35.

51. Planellas M, Cuenca R, Tabar MD, et al. Evaluation of C-reactive protein, haptoglobin and cardiac troponin 1 levels in brachycephalic dogs with upper airway obstructive syndrome. BMC Vet Res 2012;8:152–5.

52. Oginska O, Hughes J, Liu N-C, et al. An incompletely erupted canine tooth compromising the nasal cavity in a pug presenting with severe brachycephalic obstructive airway syndrome. Vet Rec Case Rep 2020;8:E000972.

53. Colberg VT, Kudej RK, Czajkowski PS, et al. Evaluation of reduction glossoplasty on airway resistance and cross-sectional areas of the upper airway in brachycephalic dogs: a cadaveric study. Chicago, Illinois: Paper presented at: 2021 American College of Veterinary Surgeons Surgery Summit; 2021.

54. Schuenemann R, Pohl S, GU R Oechtering. A novel approach to brachycephalic syndrome. 3. Isolated laser-assisted turbinectomy of caudal aberrant turbinates (CAT LATE). Vet Surg 2017;46:32–8.

55. Topfer T, Kohler C, Rosch S, et al. Brachycephaly in French bulldogs and pugs is associated with narrow ear canals. Vet Dermatol 2022;33:214-e60.

56. Tobias KM, Jackson AM, Harvey RC. Effects of doxapram HCl on laryngeal function of normal dogs and dogs with naturally occurring laryngeal paralysis. Vet Anes and Analgesia 2004;31(4):258–63.

57. Sakai DM, Howard SL, Reed RA, et al. Influence of doxapram and intermittent 10% carbon dioxide inspiration on cardiovascular and laryngeal functions in anesthetized dogs. Vet Surg 2021;50:1418–26.

58. Kossa MC, Yu Y, Hey J, et al. Pharmacological characterization of a noninvasive, chronic, experimental dog model of nasal congestion. J Pharmacol Toxicol Methods 2002;47:11–7.

59. Franklin PH, Liu N-C, Ladlow JF. Nebulization of epinephrine to reduce severity of brachycephalic obstructive airway syndrome in dogs. Vet Surg 2021;50:62–70.

60. Grosso OF Vilaplana, Ter Haar G, Boroffka SAEB. Gender, weight, and age effects on prevalence of caudal aberrant nasal turbinates in clinically healthy English bulldogs: A computed tomographic study and classification. Vet Radiol Ultrasound 2015;56(5):486–93.

61. Schmidt-Nielsen K, Bretz WL, Taylor CR. Panting in dogs: Unidirectional air flow over evaporative surfaces. Science 1970;169:1102–4.

62. GU Oechtering. Diseases of the nose, sinuses and nasopharynx. In: Ettinger SJ, Feldman EC, Cote E, editors. Textbook of veterinary internal medicine. 8th ed. Philadelphia, PA: Elsevier; 2017. p. 1059–76.

63. Lorinson D, Bright RM, White RAS. Brachycephalic airway obstructive syndrome- a review of 118 cases. Canine Pract 1997;22:18–21.

64. Dunie-Merigot A, Bouvy B, Poncet C. Comparative use of CO2 laser, diode laser, and monopolar electrocautery for resection of the soft palate in dogs with brachycephalic airway obstructive syndrome. Vet Rec 2010;167:700–4.

65. Worth DB, Grimes JA, Jiménez DA, et al. Risk factors for temporary tracheostomy tube placement following surgery to alleviate signs of brachycephalic obstructive airway syndrome in dogs. J Am Vet Med Assoc 2018;253(9):1158–63.

66. Sanuki T, Mishima G, Ayuse T. Effect of dexmedetomidine sedation on swallowing reflex: A pilot study. J Dent Sci 2020;15(2):207–13.

Laser-Assisted Retropharyngeal Rigid Nasopharyngoscopy in Dogs

Boel A. Fransson, DVM, PhD, DACVS*

KEYWORDS

- Pharyngoscopy • Rigid endoscopy • Laser-assisted surgery

KEY POINTS

- Retrograde rigid nasopharyngoscopy provides access for endoscope with operative sheath and 5-mm instruments into the nasopharynx, allowing for effective but piecemeal marginal resection of masses.
- The approach is primarily diagnostic but can have therapeutic benefits if the mass is confined to the nasopharynx.
- Hemorrhage affecting endoscopic visualization is the main intraoperative complication.
- The surgical recoveries in three large-breed mesocephalic dogs were uneventful with minimal pain and no overt complications. The dogs were ready for discharge from the hospital the following morning.

Access to the nasopharynx in dogs and cats has been gained through several approaches: open surgery by retraction or incision of the soft palate, oral retroflexed endoscopy, retroesophageal nasopharyngoscopy, and normograde rhinoscopy. All approaches have distinct advantages and disadvantages. This article discusses various approaches to nasopharynx of small animals and introduces early results of a novel approach with rigid endoscopy for laser resection or ablation of tumors in this anatomic region.

ORAL APPROACHES TO THE PHARYNX AND NASOPHARYNX

Traditionally the nasopharynx in canine and feline patients have been approached noninvasively by retraction of the soft palate or invasively by a full-thickness incision through the palatine tissues.[1] Retraction of the soft palate provides limited visualization and is mainly used for benign lesions. In this author's experience palate retraction is an excellent approach for foreign body retrieval or traction avulsion of single

Department of Veterinary Clinical Sciences, College of Veterinary Medicine, Washington State University, Pullman, WA 99164, USA
* Corresponding author.
E-mail address: boel_fransson@wsu.edu

Vet Clin Small Anim 54 (2024) 637–647
https://doi.org/10.1016/j.cvsm.2024.02.012
0195-5616/24/© 2024 Elsevier Inc. All rights reserved.

vetsmall.theclinics.com

nasopharyngeal polyps if the lesion is large and caudally located. These types of lesions are often easily palpable through the soft palate. If small or cranially located, palpation seldom reveals the lesion and palate retraction usually fails to visualize it.

Open surgical approaches include ventral midline rhinotomy for the cranial nasopharynx and nasopharyngeal approach for central pharyngeal or caudal nasopharyngeal lesions.[1] The invasiveness of these approaches leads to risks for several complications. For the ventral rhinotomy especially, stricture of the nasopharynx is associated with aggressive surgical debridement.[1] Severe hemorrhage is a risk with the highly vascular tissues in the nasal passages, and cats with hemostasis attempted by carotid artery tourniquets have died as a result.[2] Meticulous suturing ideally in three layers is required to overcome the incisional tension caused by tensor palatine muscles.[1] Suturing in thin soft palates under limited visualization due to location is challenging, and oronasal fistula has been reported as a complication.[2] Apart from complications the traditional approaches limit the visual field of the nasopharynx. Visualization cranial to the incision is not provided.

ENDOSCOPIC APPROACHES TO THE NASOPHARYNX

To overcome the risks and poor visualization of traditional surgery several minimally invasive approaches have been described.

Normograde and Retroflexed Nasopharyngoscopy

Normograde (anterior) rigid rhinoscopy can visualize nasopharynx mainly in medium to large-breed dogs. However, the small size of the osseous choana limits the degrees of freedom of scope manipulation even in larger breed dogs, especially if an operative sheath is needed for electrosurgical hemostasis; this makes manipulation of lesions dorsal or ventral to the immediate axis of the rigid scope challenging. In small breed dogs or cats, nasopharyngeal access from anterior rhinoscopy is possible with small rigid scopes without an operative sheet, in combination with visualization from retroflexed endoscopy.[3] Recently traction-avulsion of small middle ear polyps was successfully demonstrated in five cats, using this rigid and flexible endoscopy combination.[3] Highly vascularized, larger, or more caudally located masses in the nasopharynx are likely challenging to address this way, as the lack of an operative sheath prohibits use of laser or electrocautery hemostasis. For such lesions oral retroflexed endoscopy using flexible scopes have been used for diagnostic and therapeutic access.[4,5] Although demonstrated to be very helpful when used by experienced endoscopists,[5] the retroflexed endoscopy approach shows several limitations. The small pharyngeal cavity in many dogs and cats limits the size of scope, making the working channel size small. Thus, only very small instruments are possible to use, sometimes precluding therapeutic intervention. In addition, interference with the endotracheal tube, difficulty manipulating the endoscope and instruments, difficulty keeping the camera centered in the nasopharynx, and suboptimal image quality have been noted.[3,6]

Retrograde Flexible Nasopharyngoscopy

The challenges of retroflexed endoscopy in cats prompted two different retrograde approaches for flexible endoscopy of the nasopharynx in cats. A retrograde gastroesophageal access to the nasopharynx was reported in a cat,[7] and a retroesophagoscopic approach was demonstrated in 36 feline cadavers and 2 live cats.[6] The gastroesophageal access was performed after multiple attempts to remove nasal polyps in a cat by retroflexed endoscopy had failed. The access to the nasopharynx was achieved by a conventional gastrotomy requiring a ventral midline celiotomy that limits the minimal invasiveness of the procedure.[7] However, the retrograde approach allowed a much bigger flexible scope to be used than by retroflexed nasopharyngoscopy. The authors commented on the easier use of instruments and the improved instrument control as compared with traditional retroflexed endoscopy.[7]

The retroesophagoscopic approach was performed by inserting right-angle forceps orally extending into the proximal esophagus, providing lateral pressure on the forceps until they bluntly penetrated the esophageal wall and was visualized through a small stab incision in the skin.[6] The forceps grasped a protective cap (the flared end of a red rubber tube) into which the flexible scope was inserted and by traction moved the cap and scope into the oral cavity, for subsequent scope redirection into the nasopharynx. The surgical approach was thus very similar to the first steps of the commonly performed esophageal feeding tube placement. In comparison with traditional retroflexed endoscopy, the approach offered easier and faster visualization of the nasopharynx among inexperienced veterinarians and larger instruments for manipulation.[6] However, the cadaveric part of the study was experimental, and the technique was used therapeutically in only one cat with a quick foreign body removal, so more extensive investigations are needed to see how this technique would perform in resection of larger neoplastic lesions.

Retropharyngeal Rigid Nasopharyngoscopy for Mass Removal in Dogs

Because of the limitations of instrumentation and visualization offered by retroflexed nasopharyngoscopy we recently started to approach neoplastic lesions by a novel approach. Inspired by the encouraging results of the retroesophageal approach in cats,[5] the oncology and surgical team found it likely that a retropharyngeal approach would gain similar advantages if used in large-breed dolicho- or mesaticephalic dogs. In dogs with large neoplastic lesions in the cranial nasopharynx, a normograde rhinoscopy approach is another option. However, with a tumor obstructing visualization and causing anatomic changes, we suspected the risk for iatrogenic trauma to the ethmoid cribriform plate with possible neurologic complications would increase. The maneuverability of the scope and laser wand through the operative sheet has also been limited in our experience of normograde rhinoscopy. We therefore proceeded with retropharyngeal nasopharyngoscopy in a series of 3 dogs.

CASE SERIES
Case 1

A 12-year-old male castrated border collie presented for evaluation of a nasopharyngeal mass. History included dyspnea and progressive stertor for 2 months. Before evaluation at our institution a computed tomographic (CT) scan demonstrated a soft-tissue attenuating nasopharyngeal mass. Histopathological examination interpreted the mass as being poorly differentiated and likely of mesenchymal origin, but carcinoma could not be ruled out. On presentation to our institution the previous clinical signs remained, including halitosis with foul odor. A minimal data basis (complete blood count [CBC], chemistry profile) and thoracic radiographs were within normal limits. On contrast CT, a 26 mm × 26 mm heterogeneously contrast-enhancing soft tissue mass was noted to occlude the nasopharynx (**Fig. 1A**).

The dog returned for surgical treatment 1 week later. Anesthesia was routine with endotracheal intubation and use of 100% oxygen for anesthetic gas delivery. The cuff on the endotracheal tube was kept securely inflated throughout the procedure to protect the airway from blood and to minimize oxygen leakage into the oral cavity.

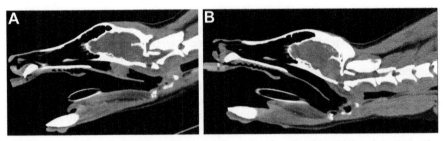

Fig. 1. Computerized tomography (CT) in case number 1; a 12-year-old border collie with a nasopharyngeal adenocarcinoma. (*A*) CT before surgery and (*B*) CT 8 months after surgery and 6 months post-radiation therapy.

The dog was placed in left lateral recumbency and the lateral laryngeal and pharyngeal region prepared and draped for aseptic surgery. A laparoscopic probe was inserted into the mouth and directed caudal to the dorsal pharyngeal region, into an area considered safe for portal placement based on historical pharyngostomy tube placement (**Fig. 2**). The probe was directed laterally to place the buccal tissue and skin under tension, and a 20-mm incision was made over the tip of the probe. An 11-mm threaded reuseable cannula (EndoTIP, Karl Storz, Goleta, CA, USA) was placed over the blunt instrument tip (**Fig. 3**). A 2.9-mm 30° rigid endoscope in a 4-mm operative sheath with 17G working channel (Stryker hysteroscope, Kalamazoo, MI, USA) was used to visualize the mass (see **Fig. 3**; **Fig. 4**) in a caudal to rostral orientation. A 600-μm diode laser fiber (AccuVet 50D 980 nm 50 W and 635 nm 4 mW diode surgical laser, AccuVet laser surgery) was introduced through the working channel in the operative sheath and used at 12 to 15 W in a continuous manner to resect the mass (see **Fig. 4**B). Hemostasis was in part achieved by the diode laser, but in part hemorrhage also had to be suctioned using an 8-Fr red rubber tube inserted in the left (dependent) nostril and continuing into the nasopharynx. Intermittently, suctioning was also performed with a pool tip in the oral cavity and through the cannula as needed. The mass was resected piece-meal, and sections of the mass were retrieved

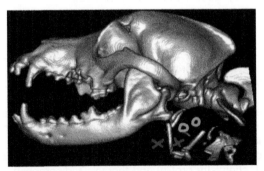

Fig. 2. Portal placements for retrograde nasopharyngoscopy. Areas considered safe for portal entry are denoted by green circles and areas considered unsafe by red X, based on previous guidelines for pharyngostomy tube placement. In this series portals were placed with the buccal tissue and overlying skin tensed by instruments inserted orally into the caudal dorsal buccal pouch, with a skin incision over the top of the instrument and portals passed either over the instrument or by the instrument pulling the portals into the oral cavity for redirection into the nasopharynx.

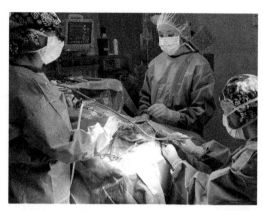

Fig. 3. Intraoperative image from case no. 1, positioned in left lateral recumbency with the head to the right in the image. A threaded 11-mm portal is inserted. A 2.9-mm 30° rigid endoscope in a 4-mm operative sheet with 17G working channel (Stryker hysteroscope, Kalamazoo, MI, USA) is directed into the nasopharynx. In the image hemorrhage is being suctioned through the oral cavity with a poole tip. Additionally, 8- to 16-Fr red rubber catheters placed nasally were used in all three cases for improved visualization.

using a 5-mm laparoscopic grasper placed side by side with the scope in the cannula. Resection was considered completed when no more visual mass remained and a patent nasopharynx with clear visualization of the choana was present (see **Fig. 4**C). The oropharyngeal defect was closed with two simple interrupted sutures via 2-0 PDS using a portal closure device/suture grasper (Progressive Medical, Inc. Fenton, MO) similar to how this device is used to close laparoscopic portals (**Fig. 5**). Muscular layers were closed extra-orally with a simple interrupted suture pattern using 3-0 PDS. The subcutaneous tissue and dermis were closed using two buried simple interrupted 3-0 monocryl sutures. Bupivacaine liposome local anesthetic (Nocita, Elanco US, Greenfield, IN, USA) was administered intraincisionally into the surrounding subcutaneous tissue and deep into the surrounding muscles. There was moderate right-sided swelling of the oropharyngeal cavity during closure but without clinical evidence of airway obstruction. One dose of dexamethasone sodium phosphate was given to decrease the risk for airway swelling.

The dog recovered in the intensive care unit receiving analgesia (methadone and gabapentin), a proton pump inhibitor (pantoprazole), and an antiemetic (maropitant), and the surgical site was cold compressed every 6 hours. The recovery was

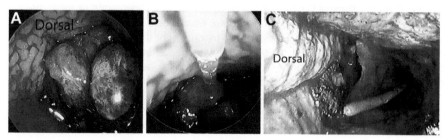

Fig. 4. Intraoperative images of case 1. (*A*) A friable and hemorrhagic mass was visualized in mid-nasopharynx. (*B*) A diode laser handpiece is directed toward the suspected attachment of the mass. (*C*) After completed resection, the nasopharynx is patent with all visible tumor removed, and a red rubber catheter is seen protruding from the choana.

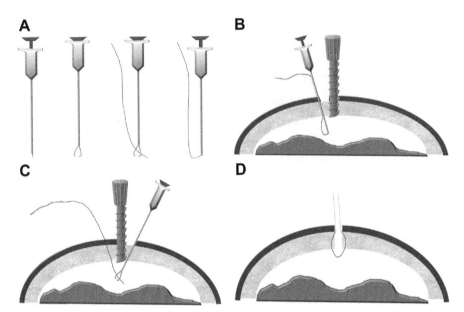

Fig. 5. Steps for suturing portal sites utilizing a portal closure device (PCD) as in case 1. (*A*) The needlescopic instrument exteriorizes a grasper when the blue button is pressed. The suture is grasped and with the button released pulled into the needle shaft. (*B*) The PCD is inserted into the skin incision lateral to the portal, and the suture is released by pressing the button. (*C*) The PCD is inserted on the contralateral side of the portal, and the suture is regrasped. (*D*) After withdrawing the PCD the portal site suture can be tied.

uneventful, and the following day the dog was comfortable on oral gabapentin, was eating canned food well, and drinking water normally. The dog was discharged from the hospital the day after surgery.

The histologic diagnosis was nasopharyngeal adenocarcinoma, and surgical margins were considered incomplete as expected.

The dog returned to the hospital 2 weeks later for radiation therapy (RT). A CT performed for RT showed no evidence of tumor, and the dog was treated with 10 fractions of 4.2 Gy administered daily over 10 consecutive working days.

The dog returned to the hospital for two follow-up consultations 5 months and 8 months after surgery. There were no descriptions of RT adverse effects or signs of stertor or nasal discharge since completion of RT. The dog was described as clinically normal at home. Repeat CT of head and thorax did not show signs of local disease recurrence or metastasis (**Fig. 1**B). Retroflex endoscopic examination did not show signs of local tumor regrowth. However, 10 months after the initial presentation to our hospital the dog showed signs of lethargy and inappetence. Evaluation revealed pericardial and peritoneal effusion with several splenic nodules but no obvious right atrial or auricular mass; pericardiocentesis obtained hemorrhagic fluid without evidence of neoplastic cells or infectious organisms. Two days later the dog died at home, presumably from recurrence of pericardial effusion. A necropsy was not performed. Before the dog's death, there were no clinical signs of nasopharyngeal disease.

Case 2

A 2.5-year-old female spayed German short-haired pointer and Labrador mix was presented to our institution for evaluation of a nasopharyngeal mass. Three months earlier the dog had been seen at the referring DVM for nasal congestion, sneezing, and ocular discharge. Corticosteroids (trimeprazine with prednisolone) and clindamycin had been prescribed but as the dog did not improve, these medications were discontinued, and amoxicillin/clavulanic acid was initiated. Two months later the dog had developed a mass above her left eye that was painful to touch. In addition, two events of left-sided epistaxis had been noted. Thoracic radiographs and blood work were unremarkable. Skull radiographs revealed lysis over the left portion of the frontal bone. Endoscopy revealed a vascularized nasopharyngeal mass.

The dog was presented to the oncology service at our institution, and a contrast CT was performed (**Fig. 6**A). Conclusions included an extensive left nasal mass causing expansive regional lysis, including early extension into the cranial vault. Thoracic radiographs were within normal limits. Cytology samples obtained from the mass over her left eye showed low proliferation of mildly atypical epithelial cells and neutrophilic inflammation. Biopsies obtained through frontal sinus trephination with tissue collected from the sinus and the nasal passage were interpreted on histopathological examination as severe eosinophilic rhinitis. Fungal and bacterial cultures were negative.

Because of the discrepancy of the severity of the changes noted on CT with the benign results obtained on samples obtained from nasal cavity and frontal sinus, additional biopsies were recommended.

The dog was anesthetized, positioned, and surgically prepared similar to case 1. The skin and buccal tissue was tented using laparoscopic cobra forceps instead of the blunt probe used in case 1. The skin was incised over the tip of the grasper and the grasper bluntly pushed through the buccal tissues. The instrument grasped the end of a 16-G peel-away introducer sheath and pulled it through the incision into the oral cavity. The same rigid scope as in case 1 was used to visually inspect and redirect the sheath into the nasopharynx. A second peel-away sheath was placed adjacent to the first one and used to introduce laparoscopic grasping forceps, alternating with a 5-mm laparoscopic suctioning and irrigation device. A red rubber tube was passed in the dependent left nostril into the nasopharynx similar to case 1 to aid in visualization by removing hemorrhage.

All visual mass in the nasopharynx (**Fig. 6**B) was removed using diode laser, biopsy forceps, and graspers as needed. The procedure was considered complete when the nasopharynx was patent and choanae visualized (**Fig. 6**C). A 5-mm laparoscopic suction tip was passed through the left nasal passage until visualized in the choana to further suction blood and aid in visualization. Peel-away sheets were removed without suturing the defects. The oral cavity was suctioned before extubation to remove blood and lavage fluid.

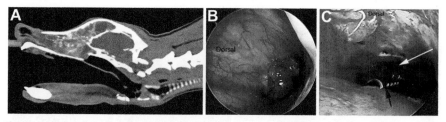

Fig. 6. Case 2; a 2.5-year-old (large) mixed breed with eosinophilic rhinitis/sinusitis and lysis of bone before surgery. (*A*) CT of the mass preoperatively. (*B*) The mass is protruding from the nasal cavity into the proximal nasopharynx. (*C*) The visible mass has been removed for biopsy (*white arrow* at previous tumor location). A 5-mm laparoscopic suctioning tip (*black arrow*) is protruding from the left choana. *Asterix* indicates small swelling from trauma associated with portal and does not represent tumor.

The dog recovered uneventfully and received firocoxib and gabapentin for analgesia, as well as antianxiety medication (trazodone) and antiemetics (maropitant), and was discharged from the hospital the day after the procedure.

Biopsies were composed of well-differentiated bone and granulation tissue considered reactive tissue as well as tissue diagnosed as eosinophilic rhinitis. The dog was lost to follow-up.

Case 3

A 10-year-old male castrated border collie was presented to our oncology service for further evaluation of a suspected nasal tumor in the left nasal passage. Twelve weeks earlier the dog had been seen by the referring DVM for evaluation of purulent nasal discharge, difficulty breathing during the night, and frequent sneezing. Amoxicillin/clavulanic acid was prescribed, and the clinical signs subsided for about a week, whereafter the dog became more lethargic and showed progressive dyspnea. One month later nasal cytology and culture indicated suppurative inflammation and the presence of mycoplasma, respectively. The antibiotic was changed to doxycycline. Six weeks later a CT scan showed that the cribriform plate and ethmoid turbinates were obscured by fluid, and the dog was referred to our hospital.

Thoracic radiographs were within normal limits. A contrast CT demonstrated a focally destructive mass in the left nasal passage and rostral nasopharynx with ipsilateral rhinitis (**Fig. 7**A) but no regional lymphadenomegaly. Biopsies obtained without visual guidance through the left nasal passage demonstrated neutrophilic mucinous exudate with hemorrhage.

Because of the nondiagnostic biopsies, the dog returned to the surgery service for attempting additional biopsies one month later. The dog was significantly dyspneic especially at night and showed difficulties sleeping, and the owner was questioning the dog's quality of life. Blood work (CBC, chemistry panel) and thoracic radiographs were unremarkable.

The dog was anesthetized, positioned, and surgically prepared similar to case 1 and 2 but was placed in right lateral recumbency in contrast to the previous cases.

Access to the nasopharynx was performed as in case 2, using two 16-G peel-away introducer sheets as cannulas. The cranial nasopharyngeal/choanal mass was resected similar to case 2, and hemostasis was likewise managed as in previous cases. The resection was considered complete when the choana was patent (**Fig. 7**B, C) and a 16-Fr red rubber tube could be easily passed from the nasal cavity into the nasopharynx without additional tumor visible. Cannula sites were not surgically closed and analgesia managed as in the previous cases.

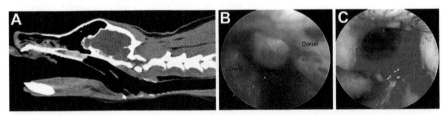

Fig. 7. Case 3; a 10-year-old border collie with nasal and proximal nasopharyngeal chondrosarcoma. (*A*) CT of the mass preoperatively. (*B*) The mass is protruding from the nasal cavity into the proximal nasopharynx. (*C*) The visible mass has been removed for biopsy. One of the 16-G peel-away sheets used as cannulas is visible in the lower left corner.

The dog initially recovered with dysphoria and hypoxia and was reintubated and provided oxygen. Thirty minutes later he was reextubated and recovered uneventfully with mild epistaxis and mild swelling at the cannula sites. He was discharged from the hospital the day after the procedure at which time he was bright, alert, and was eating well.

The biopsies were histologically diagnosed as a chondroid neoplasm, presumptively chondrosarcoma. Because of the absence of mitotic figures and binucleated cells within the chondroid matrix, differentiation from chondroma was difficult but a sarcoma was suspected based on the CT-reported invasion of the maxilla.

The owner declined additional treatment, and after communication regarding the histopathological diagnosis the dog was lost to follow-up.

SURGICAL DISCUSSION

The three cases discussed here were all undergoing retrograde rigid nasopharyngoscopy through a retropharyngeal approach for laser ablation of presumed neoplasia. The access sites were based on historical reports on safe versus unsafe sites for pharyngostomy tube placement (see **Fig. 2**).[8] In all cases the procedures were presented to the owners as primarily of diagnostic value. However, case 1 with an obstructive mid-nasopharyngeal mass in addition gained almost 10 months of palliation from clinical signs. The two latter cases did not receive the same palliative benefits. Case 2 had extensive remaining disease in the nasal cavity and sinus that the retrograde approach was unable to treat. Case 3 had a mass located in the caudal nasal cavity as well as into the choana and proximal nasopharynx. Despite the procedure seemingly obtaining a patent airway, the small lumen of the surgical site, combined with surgical trauma and likely residual nasal tumor, was precluding the dog to regain airflow through the affected nostril during the first 10 days after the procedure. Unfortunately, both case 2 and 3 were lost to follow-up after conversations with the owners regarding histologic diagnosis.

The combined experiences from these cases show that the procedure can be expected to provide diagnostic samples if a mass is located in the nasopharynx. Therapeutic benefits may be obtained if the mass is confined to the nasopharynx and not extending into the choana and the nasal passage or beyond.

The retrograde approach shows several advantages and some disadvantages compared with other endoscopic approaches. Compared with retroflexed endoscopy, surgical manipulation and visualization seems greatly aided by the ability to use instruments that can provide larger grasping capabilities than the working channel in the flexible scopes admits. Visualization and manipulation has also been demonstrated to be improved in a retrograde as compared with a retroflexed endoscopic approach.[6] Normograde rhinoscopy can also provide access to the nasopharynx, but resection of larger nasopharyngeal masses is limited by the reduced freedom of movement the narrow choanal passage provides. However, it is possible that case 2 and 3 could have benefitted from additional tumor resection from a normograde approach. A normograde approach was not chosen in case 2, as the complete obstruction of the nasal passage paired with destruction of the cranial vault seemed associated with risks for poor visualization and potential neurologic complications.

The retrograde approach is more invasive than a retroflexed or normograde approach. However, all three dogs in this short series recovered with no detectable pain, minimal epistaxis, or other clinical signs. Because of the uncomplicated recovery all three dogs were ready for discharge the morning after the procedure. Hemorrhage during and after the procedures was not significant enough to cause anemia, and the packed cell volumes postoperatively were similar to preoperative values or only mildly decreased in all three cases.

The surgical technique was modified from case 1 to the subsequent cases. In the first case one larger cannula was used in contrast to cases 2 and 3 where two smaller peel-away sheets were used. The modification was done to avoid having to suture the cannula defect. It is unknown whether suturing of the cannula site in the first dog was necessary, but with a relatively sizable defect in the caudal pharynx we considered it safer to close the defect than to allow it for second intention healing. Case 2 and 3 with the two smaller cannulas did not show any problems from their pharyngeal defects that healed by second intention. Laparoscopic graspers were advantageous when placing the softer peel-away sheets, as they could pull the sheath with its dilator into the oral cavity and then the system could be relocated into the nasopharynx. Peel-away sheets are designed for vascular or nonvascular introduction. However, to push large sheaths through the buccal tissues, as opposed to pulling them, seems difficult due to the relatively limited landing zone of the nasopharynx and risk for inadvertent trauma to structures including the mass.

A major challenge of approaching nasopharyngeal masses endoscopically is the associated bleeding. Hemorrhage was subjectively the main cause of limitations to visualization in these cases. Laser ablation was not able to completely prevent hemorrhage, as anticipated. Hemorrhage was managed by suctioning through a normograde catheter placed in the dependent nasal cavity. Therefore, the dog was positioned such that the ipsilateral side of the mass in case 2 and 3 was placed in the nondependent position. Toward the end of the procedure another tube was placed in the ipsilateral nostril to aid in suction and to demonstrate a patent choana. Despite the bleeding, the visible nasopharyngeal masses were resectable in all three cases presented here.

In conclusion, retrograde rigid nasopharyngoscopy through a retropharyngeal approach showed significant potential, especially in masses confined to the nasopharynx. The biggest complications included visualization problems associated with surgical trauma to these highly hemorrhagic masses. This approach warrants further evaluation in additional cases and in breeds with other nasal conformations than those presented here.

CLINICS CARE POINTS

- A number of minimally invasive approaches are available for access to nasal passages and nasopharynx.
- For therapeutic access a retrograde approach seems to carry several advantages.
- Control of hemorrhage is needed for optimal visualization, and a combination of suctioning and laser use for tumor resection was helpful in this respect.

DISCLOSURE

The author has no conflicts of interest to report. The work was not funded.

REFERENCES

1. Weeden AM, Degner DA. Surgical Approaches to the Nasal Cavity and Sinuses. Vet Clin North Am Small Anim Pract 2016;46:719–33.

2. Holmberg DL. Sequelae of ventral rhinotomy in dogs and cats with inflammatory and neoplastic nasal pathology: a retrospective study. Can Vet J 1996;37:483–5.

3. Oorsprong CW, Ter Haar G. Rigid normograde rhinoscopy-assisted traction-avulsion removal of small middle ear polyps from the auditory tube in five cats. J Feline Med Surg 2023;25. 1098612X231179077.

4. Hunt GB, Perkins MC, Foster SF, et al. Nasopharyngeal disorders of dogs and cats: A review and retrospective study. Compend Continuing Educ Pract Vet 2002;24:184 -+.

5. De Lorenzi D, Bertoncello D, Mantovani C, et al. Nasopharyngeal sialoceles in 11 brachycephalic dogs. Vet Surg 2018;47:431–8.

6. Derre MG, Snead EC, Beaufrere HH, et al. Investigation of a retroesophagoscopic approach to nasopharyngoscopy as an alternative to the conventional retroflexed endoscopic approach for selected indications in feline cadavers and client-owned cats. Am J Vet Res 2021;82:752–9.

7. Esterline ML, Radlinsky MG, Schermerhorn T. Endoscopic removal of nasal polyps in a cat using a novel surgical approach. J Feline Med Surg 2005;7:121–4.

8. Armstrong PJ, Hand MS, Frederick GS. Enteral nutrition by tube. Vet Clin North Am Small Anim Pract 1990;20:237–75.

Laparoscopic Treatment of Sliding Hiatal Hernia

Sarah Marvel, DVM, MS, DACVS-SA[a],*, Eric Monnet, DVM, PhD, DACVS[b]

KEYWORDS

• Laparoscopy • Hiatal hernia • Brachycephalic

KEY POINTS

- Laparoscopic hiatal hernia repair is an advanced laparoscopic procedure that includes plication of the esophageal hiatus, esophagopexy, and left sided gastropexy.
- Conversion during laparoscopic repair of hiatal hernia may be indicated if visualization of the hiatus is limited, reduction of the hernia is unsuccessful, or pneumothorax occurs that cannot be rapidly treated with percutaneous drainage.
- Surgery results in improvement of clinical signs for most dogs, but in some cases the frequency of sliding hiatal hernia is unchanged or in rare cases can worsen.
- Medical management both preoperatively and postoperatively is an important adjuvant to surgery and most commonly consists of omeprazole, cisapride, ± sucralfate, and a low-fat diet.

 Video content accompanies this article at http://www.vetsmall.theclinics.com.

INTRODUCTION

Hiatal hernias involve displacement of the lower esophageal sphincter, the cardia, and in some cases the fundus of the stomach through the esophageal hiatus into the thoracic cavity. These hernias are typically sliding in dogs meaning that with changes in pressure the lower esophageal sphincter moves back and forth from the peritoneal cavity to the thoracic cavity. Congenital hiatal hernias have been reported in dogs,[1–3] but the majority are secondary to significant intrathoracic pressure changes that result from upper airway obstruction commonly seen in brachycephalic breeds.[4–7] While small sliding hiatal hernias (SHH) may be associated with mild or intermittent clinical signs that can be managed medically, larger hernias can lead to significant gastroesophageal reflux that is refractory or incompletely responds to medical management.

[a] ACVS Fellow, Surgical Oncology and MIS (SA Soft Tissue), Department of Clinical Sciences, Colorado State University, Fort Collins, CO, USA; [b] ACVS Founding Fellow, MIS (SA Soft Tissue), Department of Clinical Sciences, Colorado State University, Fort Collins, CO, USA
* Corresponding author. Colorado State University, 300 West Drake Road, Fort Collins, CO 80523.
E-mail address: Sarah.marvel@colostate.edu

Vet Clin Small Anim 54 (2024) 649–659
https://doi.org/10.1016/j.cvsm.2024.02.009
0195-5616/24/Published by Elsevier Inc.

vetsmall.theclinics.com

Treatment with an open surgical approach has been the standard of care for those that have failed medical management. The most common surgical techniques include combinations of hiatal plication (phrenoplasty), esophagopexy, and left-sided fundic gastropexy.[1–8]

In a systematic review and meta-analysis in people, laparoscopic treatment of hiatal hernia has been shown to be a safe and effective alternative to laparotomy.[9] Those that underwent laparoscopic treatment had faster convalescence, better control of long-term reflux symptoms, and lower risk of complications.[9] Laparoscopic treatment of hiatal hernia has been described in dogs.[5,6,8] While there are no prospective studies comparing laparoscopy versus laparotomy in companion animals for treatment of hiatal hernia, complications and outcomes with laparoscopy appear comparable to open surgery,[5,6,8] and presumably the same short-term benefits derived from a minimally invasive approach in people with hiatal hernia repair should apply to companion animals.

Clinical Presentation

Clinical signs associated with hiatal hernias result from gastroesophageal reflux and include regurgitation, salivation, vomiting, dysphagia, anorexia, and weight loss. Animals are at increased risk of aspiration pneumonia and may also present with lower airway signs or respiratory distress. Dogs with congenital sliding hiatal hernias typically present within ages of 2 to 4 months.[1,2] Those with acquired hernias or hernias that are worsened by an upper airway obstruction can present later in life. While a variety of clinical signs can be seen, the most common clinical sign is regurgitation, but in some cases this regurgitation can be silent and more difficult to detect. Dogs with silent regurgitation may show lip smacking, hard swallowing, or present with recurrent aspiration pneumonia. Physical examination findings are often unremarkable, but in severe cases may reveal ill thrift and low body condition score.

Diagnostics

Given the dynamic nature of sliding hiatal hernias, diagnosis can be challenging and may require multiple forms of imaging.

- *Plain thoracic radiographs* may show a stomach displaced into the thoracic cavity, but has poor sensitivity for detecting SHH (**Fig. 1**).[4,7]

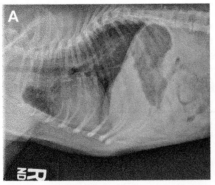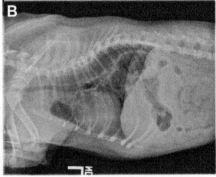

Fig. 1. A right and left lateral radiograph performed simultaneously on a brachycephalic patient. The stomach is positioned normally within the abdomen on the right lateral radiograph (*A*). The stomach is displaced into the thorax on the left lateral radiograph confirming sliding hiatal hernia (*B*).

- *Positive contrast esophagography with videofluoroscopy* is the gold standard for diagnosing dysphagia in dogs.[10] In people videofluoroscopy has been shown in multiple studies to have poor sensitivity for diagnosing SHH.[11,12] In dogs it also appears to have limitations due to the dynamic nature of SHH.[4] Despite its limitations, this is often the diagnostic of choice for identification of SHH since it can be performed in a conscious patient with normal airway pressures (unlike endoscopy) and can capture episodic events. A recent study found 44% prevalence of SHH in dogs presenting for brachycephalic obstructive airway syndrome (BOAS) surgery using videofluoroscopy, and 76% of French bulldogs had evidence of SHH.[13]
- *Endoscopy* of the esophagus and stomach has been used to document mucosal changes associated with gastroesophageal reflux, to rule out esophageal stricture as a consequence or cause of chronic regurgitation and to visualize cranial displacement of the lower esophageal sphincter.[14–16] One challenge of endoscopy is that patients are anesthetized and intubated, eliminating the upper respiratory obstructive component, which may contribute to visualizing SHH, thus leading to false negatives. A study by Broux and colleagues,[16] found that applying manual pressure on the cranial abdomen allowed detection of SHH in more dogs, however, not all dogs had gastrointestinal (GI) signs and false positives may have occurred. Other manual manipulations that may improve accuracy for detection of gastroesophageal junction abnormalities include temporary complete endotracheal tube obstruction.[16]
- *High-resolution Manometry* has been shown in people to have improved diagnostic accuracy for SHH compared to endoscopy and videofluoroscopy with positive contrast, but is not readily available in veterinary medicine.[17]

Treatment

There are currently no guidelines published in veterinary medicine to guide decision making for medical versus surgical management of patients with SHH. It is generally thought that patients with mild GI clinical signs may respond to upper airway surgery (if indicated) and/or medical management to control their symptoms. Surgery to correct the SHH should be considered in those with moderate to severe GI signs, those that are refractory to medical management, or in cases, where compliance with life-long medication is poor.

Medical management

Medical management is aimed at decreasing the acidity of the stomach to protect the esophageal mucosa when reflux occurs and improving motility of the stomach. Prescribed medications often include a combination of a proton pump inhibitor or type-2 histamine blocker and prokinetic. In some cases, mucosal protectants like sucralfate may also be recommended. A 30 day trial is often instituted to determine whether or not medical management is successful. It is important to remember that chronic use of antacid medications should be tapered prior to discontinuing.

- *Histamine type-2 receptor antagonists* like famotidine and ranitidine work by competitively blocking H-2 receptors on gastric parietal cells, suppressing gastric acid secretion. Their efficacy is considered weak compared to proton pump inhibitors (PPI) and often PPIs are preferred.
- *Proton pump inhibitors* like omeprazole and pantoprazole work by binding to the active H^+-K^+-ATPase. The efficacy of PPIs is thought to be better than H-2 receptor antagonists, but therapy with oral formulations takes a few days to reach optimal inhibitory effects, so intravenous formulations initially are recommended.

- *Cisapride* improves GI motility by acting on serotonin receptors, resulting in increased tone of the lower esophageal sphincter and improved gastric emptying. It is often administered 30 minutes prior to eating to maximize the effect. In one study, administration of cisapride in combination with a PPI, was more effective than a PPI alone at decreasing gastroesophageal reflux in anesthetized dogs undergoing elective orthopedic procedures.[18]

Surgical management

Surgical management of SHH involves a combination of procedures aimed at decreasing the size of the esophageal hiatus with a phrenoplasty and preventing the stomach from displacing into the thoracic cavity by fixing it in the abdomen with an esophagopexy and/or left sided gastropexy. In people with gastroesophageal reflux a fundoplication is often used, but outcomes in dogs with this procedure are not as successful and it appears to be associated with a higher risk of complications.[7] An open approach has traditionally been described in companion animals via a ventral midline laparotomy. A laparoscopic approach has recently been described.[5,6,8] There are still relatively few reports of laparoscopic hiatal hernia repair with some variations in patient positioning and cannula placement.

Patient positioning and cannula placement. The authors prefer the patient to be positioned in a right lateral oblique recumbancy with the left pelvic limb pulled caudally (**Fig. 2**). (Monnet 2021) The patient can also be placed in dorsal recumbency and then tilted into a right oblique position once pneumoperitoneum and cannula placement have been established. A wide abdominal clip is required with the left side approaching the dorsal midline. The patient is positioned at the end of the operating table, allowing the surgeon to stand at the back of the table, and work toward the endoscopic tower positioned at the patient's head (**Fig. 3**). Reverse trendelenberg position can facilitate exposure of the hiatus. The authors prefer using a single-port access device (SILS port; Medtronic, Minneapolis, and MN) and adding 1 or 2 cannulas of 5 to 12 mm adjacent to the single-port access device. The SILS port is placed 2 cm caudal to the last rib centered between the dorsal and ventral midline. The abdomen is insufflated up to 12 mm Hg with carbon dioxide. A 5 mm 0° or 30° laparoscope is placed through one of the 5 mm cannulas of the SILS port. Two additional cannulas are placed adjacent to the SILS port as needed (see **Fig. 2**). The authors prefer a

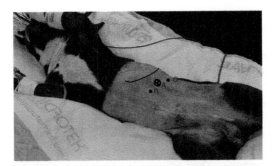

Fig. 2. The patient is positioned in right lateral recumbency with the left pelvic limb pulled caudally. A single port access device (A) is placed approximately 2 cm caudal to the last rib centered between dorsal and ventral midline. One to 2 additional cannulas (B and C) are placed adjacent to the single port access device. (*From* Monnet EM. Laparoscopic correction of sliding hiatal hernia in eight dogs: Description of technique, complications, and short-term outcome. Vet Surg. 2021;50:231.)

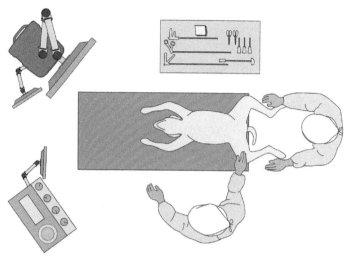

Fig. 3. Operating room setup with the patient postioned at the back end of the table to allow the surgeon to stand behind the table. The monitor is positioned near the head of the patient to allow the surgeon to work in a straight line toward the monitor. (*From* Mayhew P. Laparoscopic treatment of hiatal hernias and associated gastroesophageal reflux. In: Fransson B, Mayhew P, editors, 2nd edition. Small Animal Laparoscopy and Thoracoscopy. Hoboken, New Jersey:Wiley-Blackwell; 2022. p.159.)

5 mm cannula ventrally and a 5 to 12 mm cannula dorsally. Alternatively, a 3-port technique can be performed with the camera placed at the subumbilical site and 2 instrument cannulas, 1 on ventral midline cranial to the umbilicus and 1 in the left caudal quadrant of the abdomen (**Fig. 4**).[19]

Surgical technique. A 5 mm grasping forcep (Babcock forcep; Karl Storz, Goleta, California) is used to grasp the left triangular ligament of the liver (**Fig. 5**). Electrocautery or a bipolar vessel sealer device is then used to divide the triangular ligament (Video 1). Reduction of the lower esophageal sphincter into the abdomen is facilitated by placement of a large orogastric tube. The orogastric tube is advanced so that it sits along the greater curvature of the stomach and ends within the antrum, retracting the stomach caudally. Placement of an orogastric tube not only aids in visualization of the esophageal hiatus and lower esophageal sphincter/cardia, it also provides a guide to prevent overtightening around the lower esophageal sphincter during phrenoplasty. When hiatal hernia surgery is performed with a laparotomy the phrenicoesophageal ligament is often dissected from the esophagus. During laparoscopy, the ligament is not dissected as this seems to increase the risk of intraoperative pneumothorax.[6] Alternatively, a partial thickness thermal scar along the ventral edges of the hiatus can be performed with electrosurgery, but only if low pressure pneumoperitoneum is used (<6 mm Hg).[8] While interrupted and continuous sutures can be used, the authors prefer continuous suture pattern for technical ease. Beginning from ventral to dorsal, the esophageal hiatus is sutured. Large bites of the crural muscle on both sides of the hiatus are captured while suturing, but caution is used to avoid entering the pleural cavity. With high insufflation pressures there is a risk of carbon dioxide diffusing through the needle tracks and into the pleural space. This risk can be minimized by decreasing the insufflation pressure (4–6 mm Hg). A branch of the phrenic vein consistently lies in close proximity to the ventral hiatus and should be

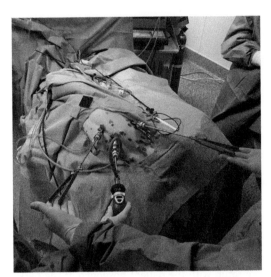

Fig. 4. Three-port technique for hiatal hernia repair with the patient tilted into right lateral recumbency. (*From* Mayhew P. Laparoscopic treatment of hiatal hernias and associated gastroesophageal reflux. In: Fransson B, Mayhew P, editors, 2nd edition. Small Animal Laparoscopy and Thoracoscopy. Hoboken, New Jersey:Wiley-Blackwell; 2022. p.160.)

avoided as well (**Fig. 6**). The authors prefer a simple continuous pattern with non-absorbable unidirectional barbed suture (VLOC PBT; Medtronic, Minneapolis, MN) using 5 mm laparoscopic needle holders (Karl Storz, **Fig. 7**) or an auto suture device (SILS-stitch or Endo-Stitch, Medtronic, Minneapolis, MN) (Video 2). Assessment of the narrowing of the esophageal hiatus is subjective, but a large orogastric tube should easily slide in and out of the stomach. The continuous suture pattern can be extended from the diaphragm to the esophagus for the esophagopexy or a new line of suture can be started (**Fig. 8**, see Video 2). Suture bites into the esophagus are partial thickness. The vagus nerve should be avoided if encountered, but often it is not visualized. Once esophagopexy is complete a left sided gastropexy can be performed. Either a left sided laparoscopic assisted or intracorporeal gastropexy is appropriate. When a single port access device is used, it is often placed at the location for gastropexy and a laparoscopic assisted gastropexy is performed through this site. Cases with severe esophagitis may benefit from temporary gastrostomy tube

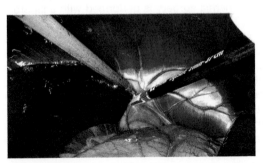

Fig. 5. A 5 mm laparoscopic babcock forcep is used to grasp the left triangular ligament to allow for transection of the left triangular ligament.

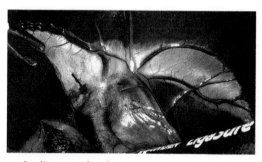

Fig. 6. The left triangular ligament has been transected to expose the esophageal hiatus. Arrow denotes the phrenic vein branch that is in close proximity to the left triangular ligament and right side of the esophageal hiatus.

placement instead of incisional gastropexy to allow the esophagus to rest in the immediate postoperative period.

Intraoperative complications and conversion

Intraoperative complications may or may not result in conversion depending on the stability of the patient and the comfort level of the surgeon. These may include minor hemorrhage either from entry techniques, reduction, or liver lobe retraction. In 1 study pneumothorax occurred in 3/8 cases.[6] Pneumothorax occurred in 1 case due to dissection of the phrenico-esophageal ligament (which was discontinued after that case) and 2 were due to needle holes from suturing the phrenoplasty. Decreasing insufflation pressures to 4 to 6 mm Hg may decrease the risk of pneumothorax secondary to suturing the diaphragm.[5,6] The surgeon should closely monitor the diaphragm while suturing. If the diaphragm loses its domed appearance and billows, rapid percutaneous thoracocentesis or thoracostomy tube placement should be performed.

Conversion rates for laparoscopic hiatal hernia repair range from 5.5% to 50%.[5,6] It is important to note that few cases of laparoscopic hiatal hernia repair have been described in the veterinary literature and therefore conversion rates are expected to be much higher earlier in the description as the technique is being modified. Conversions have been reported for both elective and emergent reasons. Elective conversions occur due to poor visualization of the hiatus from difficulty retracting the left medial and lateral liver lobes or due to difficult hernia reduction. One of the authors (EM) had 2 cases, where the papillary process of the caudate lobe was wedged into

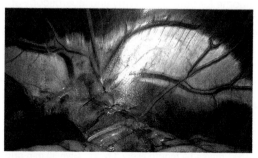

Fig. 7. Unidirectional barbed suture was used to close down the esophageal hiatus, suturing from ventral to dorsal.

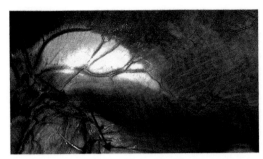

Fig. 8. Unidirecitonal barbed suture was used to complete a phrenoplasty (*black arrow*) and esophagopexy (*blue arrow*).

the hernia and attempts at reduction led to hemorrhage which obscured visualization.[6] Cardiac arrest has been reported in 2 dogs. In 1 dog conversion revealed pneumothorax, but resuscitation was not successful.[5] In the other dog the cause of cardiac arrest was unknown, conversion allowed for cardiac massage and resuscitation was successful.[6] Pneumothorax can result in rapid destabilization and may require conversion or rapid percutaneous drainage.

Postoperative Management (Patient Monitoring)

Dogs are monitored overnight in the hospital. Many of these dogs are brachycephalic and may have had concurrent upper airway surgery, so management for upper airway inflammation may be necessary. Continued management for regurgitation and/or esophagitis is typically indicated. If regurgitation occurred while anesthetized, esophageal lavage should be performed. Opioid injections and infusions may contribute to regurgitation and are used cautiously in the postoperative period. Local anesthetic injection at the port-sites may limit the amount of opioids needed in the postoperative setting. Nonsteroidal anti-inflammatories can be considered if there are no contraindications to use.

Patients are discharged on medical management for regurgitation for 2 to 4 weeks and in some cases treatment may be prolonged (**Table 1**). A low-fat diet fed in meatballs and divided into 3 to 4 meals may limit regurgitation postoperatively.

Outcomes

Information is limited on outcomes following laparoscopic hiatal hernia treatment and there are currently no prospective studies comparing laparotomy versus laparoscopy. Whilst studies on outcome for both laparotomy and laparoscopy approaches for hiatal hernia treatment are limited and outcome measures are often subjective, overall clinical outcomes appear similar. Mayhew and colleagues,[4] found that while the GI clinical signs associated with SHH improved after laparotomy to treat hiatal hernia, they did

Table 1		
Post-op medical management for continued regurgitation		
Drug	**Dosage**	**Notes**
Omeprazole	1 mg/kg by mouth every 12 h	
Cisapride	0.5–1 mg/kg by mouth every 8 h	Give 30 min prior to eating
+/− Sucralfate	1 g slurry by mouth every 8 h	Give 2 h prior to other medications

not completely resolve and videofluoroscopic swallow studies (VFSS) revealed that SHH can still persist in some patients postoperatively.[4] These are similar findings to a study performed by the same group that instead performed surgery via laparoscopy. In this study, a standardized owner assessment tool (Clinical Dysphagia Assessment Tool, CDAT) found that there was a significant decrease in the grade of regurgitation after eating and after exercise/excitement. There was also significant improvement with weight gain and ability to eat dry kibble after surgery.[5] Twelve dogs had both preoperative and postoperative VFSS for comparison and did not show any difference in frequency of esophageal dysmotility or severity, nor was there a difference in the frequency of gastroesophageal reflux. There was, however, a reduction in the severity of postoperative gastroesophageal reflux. The severity of SHH improved in 7 dogs, was unchanged in 4 dogs, and was worse in 1 dog following surgery.[5]

In a study, where 50% were converted to a laparotomy, regurgitation improved in all dogs according to the owner at a median of 16.5 days postoperatively.[6] One dog had an esophogram 2 weeks postoperatively for nausea and revealed an intact hiatus with a persistent megaesophagus. Nausea resolved with diet modification.

Therefore, overall outcomes with laparoscopy appear comparable to laparotomy. Based on VFSS some dogs may continue to have evidence of SHH after surgery, but clinical outcomes are typically improved.

DISCUSSION

Laparoscopic treatment of sliding hiatal hernia results in successful outcomes when performed by an experienced laparoscopist. Regardless of the approach performed, a multimodal diagnostic approach should occur as both false negative and false positive diagnostics can occur. Patients should undergo a medical management trial preoperatively. Surgery should be considered in those that fail to respond adequately to medical management or for those owners that are unwilling to manage medically lifelong. Surgical complications are typically managed during laparoscopy, but conversion may be needed if visualization of the hiatus is limited or reduction is unsuccessful due to adhesions. Caution should be exercised when plicating the esophagus to prevent over narrowing leading to an obstruction. Since the hiatus cannot be palpated during laparoscopy, placement of an orogastric tube can help maintain patency. Pneumothorax results from deep penetration of the phrenoplasty sutures into the pleural space coupled with high abdominal insufflation pressures which force CO_2 along the suture tracks and into the pleural space. If pneumothorax is not caught early either by detection of the diaphragm billowing or change in anesthetic parameters (tachycardia, desaturation of pulse ox, patient reacting to stimulation, etc), cardiac arrest may ensue. Rapid treatment with percutaneous drainage via a thoracostomy tube or conversion to an open laparotomy can be performed. Postoperative owner assessment reveals significant improvement in most cases. Some dogs may continue to show signs of regurgitation and gastroesophageal reflux, requiring long-term medical management. Additional prospective studies comparing laparotomy and laparoscopy for hiatal hernia repair are needed, as well as studies with more objective outcome data.

SUMMARY

Surgical treatment of hiatal hernia can be performed by laparoscopy. The surgeon should have experience in other advanced laparoscopic procedures and be familiar with intracorporeal suturing techniques. While follow-up information is limited, outcomes following laparoscopic treatment appear similar to laparotomy.

CLINICS CARE POINTS

- Surgery to correct SHH should be considered in those with moderate to severe GI signs, those that are refractory to medical management, or in cases, where compliance with life-long medication is poor.
- Positive contrast esophagography with videofluoroscopy is the gold standard for diagnosis of SHH and gastroesophageal reflux.
- Medical management is aimed at decreasing the acidity of the stomach to protect the esophageal mucosa when reflux occurs and improving the motility of the stomach.
- Positioning in an oblique right lateral recumbency during laparoscopy facilitates retraction of the liver away from the hiatus for improved visualization of the hiatal hernia.
- A large bore orogastric tube helps facilitate retraction of the stomach caudally improving visualization of the hiatus and limits overplication of the hiatus.
- Decreasing insufflation pressure to 4 to 6 mm Hg, while suturing the hiatus, limits the risk of pneumothorax.
- Rapid intraoperative thoracocentesis or thoracostomy tube placement may be needed if pneumothorax occurs.

DISCLOSURE

The authors have nothing to disclose.

SUPPLEMENTARY DATA

Supplementary data related to this article can be found online at https://doi.org/10.1016/j.cvsm.2024.02.009.

REFERENCES

1. Callan MB, Washabau RJ, Saunders HM, et al. Congenital esophageal hiatal hernia in the Chinese Shar-Pei dog. J Vet Intern Med 1993;7:210–5.
2. Guiot LP, Lansdowne JL, Rouppert P, et al. Hiatal hernia in the dog: a clinical report of four Chinese Shar-Peis. J Am Anim Hosp Assoc 2008;44:335–41.
3. Prymak C, Saunders HM, Washabau RJ. Hiatal hernia repair by restoration and stabilization of normal anatomy. An evaluation in four dogs and one cat. Vet Surg 1989;18:386–91.
4. Mayhew PD, Marks SL, Pollard R, et al. Prospective evaluation of surgical management of sliding hiatal hernia and gastroesophageal reflux in dogs. Vet Surg 2017;46:1098–109.
5. Mayhew PD, Balsa IM, Marks SL, et al. Clinical and videofluoroscopic outcomes of laparoscopic treatment for sliding hiatal hernia and associated gastroesophageal reflux in brachycephalic dogs. Vet Surg 2021;50:67–77.
6. Monnet EM. Laparoscopic correction of sliding hiatal hernia in eight dogs: Description of technique, complications, and short-term outcome. Vet Surg 2021;50:230–7.
7. Lorinson D, Bright RM. Long-term outcome of medical and surgical treatment of hiatal hernias in dogs and cats: 27 cases (1978-1996). J Am Vet Med Assoc 1998;213:381–4.
8. Cherzan NL, Fransson BA. Laparoscopic esophagopexy, fundopexy, and hiatal herniorrhaphy for refractory regurgitation in a racing alaskan husky sled dog. Can Vet J 2021;62(6):577–80.

9. Qu H, Liu Y, He QS. Short- and long-term results of laparoscopic versus open anti-reflux surgery: a systematic review and meta-analysis of randomized controlled trials. J Gastrointest Surg 2014;18:1077–86.

10. Pollard RE. Imaging evaluation of dogs and cats with dysphagia. ISRN Vet Sci 2012;238505.

11. Thompson JK, Koehler RE, Richter JE. Detection of gastroesophageal reflux: value of barium studies compared with 24-hr pH monitoring. AJR 1994;162:621–6.

12. Saleh CM, Smout AJ, Bredenoord AJ. The diagnosis of gastroesophageal reflux disease cannot be made with barium esophagrams. Neuro Gastroenterol Motil 2015;27:195–200.

13. Reeve EJ, Sutton D, Friend EJ, et al. Documenting the prevalence of hiatal hernia and oesophageal abnormalities in brachycephalic dogs using fluoroscopy. JSAP (J Small Anim Pract) 2017;58:703–8.

14. Cornell K. Stomach. In: Tobias K, Johnston S, editors. Veterinary surgery: small animal. Philadelphia: WB Saunders; 2011. p. 1500–1.

15. Washabau RJ. Disorders of the pharynx and oesophagus. In: Hall E, Simpson J, Williams D, editors. BSAVA manual of canine and Feline Gastroenterology. Gloucester, UK: BSAVA; 2005. p. 147–9.

16. Broux O, Clercx C, Etienne AL, et al. Effects of manipulations to detect sliding hiatal hernia in dogs with brachycephalic airway obstructive syndrome. Vet Surg 2018;47:243–51.

17. Kahrilas PJ, Kim HC, Pandolfino JE. Approaches to the diagnosis and grading of hiatal hernia. Best Pract Res Clin Gastroenterol 2008;22:601–16.

18. Zacuto AC, Marks SL, Osborn J, et al. The influence of esomeprazole and cisapride on gastroesophageal reflux during anesthesia in dogs. JVIM 2012;26:518–25.

19. Mayhew P. Laparoscopic treatment of hiatal hernias and associated gastroesophageal reflux. In: Fransson B, Mayhew P, editors. Small animal laparoscopy and thoracoscopy. 2nd edition. Hoboken (NJ): Wiley-Blackwell; 2022. p. 156–64.

Laparoscopic Treatment of Peritoneal-Pericardial Diaphragmatic Hernia

Valery F. Scharf, DVM, MS, DACVS*

KEYWORDS

- Laparoscopic • Peritoneal-pericardial • Hernia • Diaphragmatic • Insufflation

KEY POINTS

- Laparoscopic peritoneal-pericardial herniorrhaphy is feasible in dogs with careful case selection.
- Patients must be monitored closely for hypotension and hypoxemia secondary to pericardial and pleural insufflation, respectively.
- Abdominal insufflation should not exceed 8 mm Hg; an initial insufflation of 3 to 5 mm Hg is recommended. Tolerance of pericardial insufflation may decrease following hernia reduction. Alternatively, gasless or lift laparoscopy may be considered.
- The surgeon should be prepared for pre-emptive or emergent placement of a thoracoscopic cannula or drain in the event of tension pneumothorax.
- More research is needed to evaluate whether laparoscopic peritoneal-pericardial diaphragmatic hernia repair is safe in cats.

 Video content accompanies this article at http://www.vetsmall.theclinics.com.

CLINICAL PRESENTATION

Peritoneal-pericardial diaphragmatic hernias (PPDHs) are a relatively uncommon congenital anomaly comprising approximately 15% of diaphragmatic hernias reported in dogs and cats.[1–3] The pericardium and diaphragm in affected animals fail to form 2 distinct and complete layers separating the pericardial and peritoneal cavities. This allows for abdominal contents to herniate into the pericardial space, potentially leading to respiratory or gastrointestinal clinical signs.[1,3,4] Cats more commonly demonstrate respiratory signs, whereas dogs present more commonly with gastrointestinal signs, although as many as half of cats and dogs with PPDH do not demonstrate any clinical

Department of Clinical Sciences, NC State University, 1052 William Moore Drive, Raleigh, NC 27607, USA
* Corresponding author.
E-mail address: vfscharf@ncsu.edu

Vet Clin Small Anim 54 (2024) 661–670
https://doi.org/10.1016/j.cvsm.2024.02.003
0195-5616/24/© 2024 Elsevier Inc. All rights reserved.

signs on presentation.[1,2,4] The most commonly herniated abdominal organs include liver, gallbladder, small intestine, and omentum, although stomach, colon, falciform ligament, and spleen have also been reported.[1,3–5]

INDICATIONS AND CONTRAINDICATIONS

Surgical repair is the recommended treatment for patients presenting with clinical signs related to their PPDH. Herniorrhaphy has historically been performed via a midline celiotomy with extension to a caudal median sternotomy if indicated to dissect adhesions and facilitate reduction. Surgical treatment of aclinical cats and dogs remains controversial as the potential for sequelae to develop with age is unknown. Some advocate for repair in aclinical cats and dogs in order to minimize the risk of entrapment and strangulation of gastrointestinal viscera later in life, whereas others feel that nonclinical PPDHs do not present substantial risk of progression and therefore do not warrant the risks of herniorrhaphy unless the patient becomes clinical. Owner preference may also play a large role in determining surgical treatment in aclinical patients. Postoperative mortality rates of up to 14% have been associated with open surgical PPDH herniorrhaphy.[6] A recent retrospective study of open PPDH repair in 91 dogs found that surgical correction of PPDH was associated with low operative mortality and good long-term survival.[4] Laparoscopic PPDH herniorrhaphy may provide a useful alternative to open surgical repair.[7] A minimally invasive approach may also facilitate surgical repair in aclinical patients whose owners would prefer to avoid the morbidity of open surgery.

Appropriate case selection is critical for successful outcomes with laparoscopic PPDH repair. Extensive adhesions may make reduction more challenging and increase the likelihood of conversion. Due to the congenital nature of PPDH, adhesions may not be commonly encountered even in older patients with more chronic hernias; previous studies report adhesions in 25% or fewer of cats and dogs undergoing open surgical repair of PPDH.[1,3,4] In the author's experience, extensive adhesions appear to be more common in patients with a large proportion of the liver herniated. Unfortunately, computed tomography (CT) is of limited utility in predicting adhesions; if a large volume of liver is herniated on CT, introducing a laparoscope to first evaluate the hernia's contents before proceeding with laparoscopic repair may be prudent. Respiratory or cardiovascular compromise is considered a contraindication for laparoscopic herniorrhaphy due to the potential impacts of pericardial insufflation and the potential for pleural insufflation and hypoxemia (discussed in the following paragraphs).

DIAGNOSTICS

Thoracic radiographs may be suggestive of PPDH when an enlarged cardiac silhouette cannot be distinguished from the diaphragm on a lateral view. CT provides a much more detailed view of which organs are herniated and is recommended to help determine whether a laparoscopic approach is appropriate (**Fig. 1**). As mentioned earlier, herniation of a large portion of the liver may be associated with an increased likelihood of adhesions and more challenging reduction. Thoracic ultrasound may confirm PPDH and identify herniated organs but does not provide equivalent detail to CT. Although rare, intrapericardial cysts have been associated with PPDH; CT may also assist in identifying this intrapericardial pathology preoperatively (see **Fig. 1**) and thus aid in surgical planning.[8]

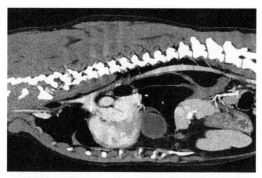

Fig. 1. Sagittal computed tomography (CT) image of a peritoneal-pericardial hernia and concurrent intrapericardial cyst. Falciform fat can be seen herniating through the ventral diaphragm into the pericardial space.

INSTRUMENTATION

Box 1 lists the relevant instrumentation for laparoscopic PPDH herniorrhaphy. The use of a suture assist device is strongly recommended due to the ability to orient the needle of the device parallel to the diaphragm which improves the ease of suturing. The author prefers to also have laparoscopic needle drivers available to facilitate the placement of a cruciate suture at the ventral aspect of the diaphragm as described earlier.

A single-incision laparoscopic surgery port may be useful to remove resected falciform fat and improve the visualization of the defect; at least 1 additional paramedian port may be needed to allow for sufficient triangulation if using laparoscopic needle drivers for intracorporeal suturing. Barbed suture is recommended to maintain tension on the herniorrhaphy and facilitate a tight, secure closure of the hernia defect.

Box 1

Instrumentation for laparoscopic peritoneal-pericardial diaphragmatic hernia herniorrhaphy

Required
- 5-mm or 10-mm 0° or 30° laparoscope
- 3 to 4 camera and instrument cannulas (unless using single incision port)
- Blunt palpation probe
- Atraumatic grasping forceps (2 pairs may be useful for reduction of fatty tissue)
- Pericardial catheter or red rubber catheter or other drain to remove pericardial insufflation
- Suture assist device or laparoscopic needle drivers

Recommended
- Barbed suture
- Vessel sealing device (to dissect adhesions)
- Hook scissors

Optional
- Fan retractor
- Metzenbaum scissors
- Lift device for gasless laparoscopy
- Single incision laparoscopic surgery port
- Thoracoscopic cannula or thoracostomy drain

SURGICAL APPROACH

A wide clip including both abdomen and thorax is indicated to allow for conversion to celiotomy and caudal median sternotomy if needed. The patient is placed in reverse Trendelenburg to facilitate reduction of viscera into the abdominal cavity (**Fig. 2**). A subumbilical camera port is placed and a 0° or 30° laparoscope introduced to visualize the hernia and confirm the extent of organ herniation (**Fig. 3**). Insufflation should be started at a maximum of 8 mm Hg and systemic blood pressure monitored closely for hypotension; the author prefers to start insufflation at 5 mm Hg and gradually increase as needed if tolerated by the patient. Once the hernia is visualized and proceeding with a laparoscopic approach is confirmed, 2 additional ports are placed in the right and left paramedian quadrants. In very large dogs, care should be taken to ensure that these ports are placed sufficiently cranial to allow laparoscopic instruments to reach the diaphragm. Resection of the falciform fat may assist in visualizing and suturing the hernia. Resected falciform fat can be removed through a single-incision laparoscopic surgery port without disrupting port incisions and interfering with insufflation; alternatively, the falciform may be removed by enlarging an instrument cannula at the end of the procedure. Moving the camera port to 1 of the paramedian ports may also improve visualization and instrument manipulation around the falciform fat.

REDUCTION

Once adhesions have been dissected, contents of the hernia are reduced through the defect. PPDH defects are usually sufficiently large such that incisions to extend the hernia are only necessary to dissect adhesions rather than to facilitate reduction. Different organs are associated with specific challenges during hernia reduction. Vessel sealers (bipolar or ultrasonic) may be useful for dissection of adhesions (Video 1). If near the surface of the heart, care should be taken to minimize the risk of fibrillation from proximity of a bipolar vessel sealer.[9] Vascular solid organs such as liver and spleen should be gently manipulated with a sweeping motion using a blunt instrument or fan retractor to minimize iatrogenic puncture and bleeding (Video 2).

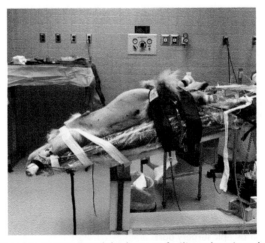

Fig. 2. A patient placed in reverse Trendelenburg to facilitate hernia reduction during laparoscopic peritoneal-pericardial diaphragmatic hernia (PPDH) herniorrhaphy.

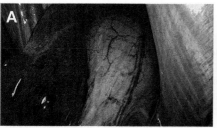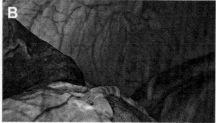

Fig. 3. The right medial liver lobe and gallbladder are shown herniating through the peritoneal-pericardial diaphragmatic hernia (PPDH) in this dog. (*A*) shows the right medial liver lobe and gallbladder herniating passing through the hernia into the pericardium. This view was obtained by placing the camera and laparoscope through the right paramedian port to minimize interference from the falciform ligament. (*B*) shows a pericardioscopic view of the liver lobe and gallbladder wall (*left*) and epicardium (*right*) within the pericardial space.

Temporarily increasing the angle of reverse Trendelenburg may be helpful to facilitate reduction of these heavy organs. Omental fat and small intestines are less dependent on gravity for reduction and may require gentle traction with a blunt probe or atraumatic grasping forceps on the omentum and mesentery. A paired set of forceps are useful to allow 1 grasper to maintain the position of the fat or intestines while the other applies additional traction in a hand-over-hand manner (Video 3). If adhesions are extensive, thoracoscopic ports may be placed in the ventral fifth through seventh intercostal spaces to facilitate thoracoscopic dissection of adhesions after opening the pericardium. If the patient tolerates pericardial insufflation, pericardioscopy can be performed following reduction to evaluate for any abnormalities (ie, intrapericardial cyst), although the ability to view the caudodorsal pericardial space may be limited by the angle of the laparoscope through the subumbilical port and hernia ring (**Fig. 4**).

HERNIORRHAPHY

Once all contents have been reduced into the abdomen, herniorrhaphy is performed by suturing from the dorsal aspect of the defect to the ventral aspect. The necessity of freshening the edges of the hernia prior to closure is unknown; the author does

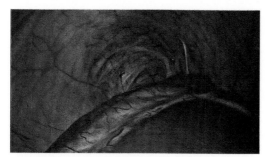

Fig. 4. Pericardioscopy shows the ventral pericardial space following peritoneal-pericardial diaphragmatic hernia (PPDH) reduction. Visualization of the dorsal pericardial space may be limited by the angle of the laparoscope. Systemic blood pressure should be carefully monitored while insufflating the pericardial space.

not routinely do this when repairing PPDH as the hernia ring may provide additional holding strength. Closure is performed in 1 or 2 layers in an interrupted or simple continuous pattern (Video 4). The use of barbed suture helps maintain tension while closing the defect. The author prefers to use a single-layer simple continuous closure with 2-0 barbed suture. The use of a suture assist device instead of traditional laparoscopic needles drivers is strongly recommended as the orientation of the needle of the suture assist device perpendicular to the diaphragm dramatically improves the ease of suturing (**Fig. 5**). Prior to complete closure of the defect, a 5-Fr red rubber catheter or pericardiocentesis catheter is passed percutaneously or through a cannula into the abdomen and then into the pericardial space (**Fig. 6**). This catheter is left in place while the remainder of the defect is closed. Negative suction is then applied as the catheter is withdrawn from the pericardial space to evacuate any gas remaining in the pericardium. Alternatively, if the pericardium was breached during reduction or herniorrhaphy, a thoracic drain can be placed to evacuate pericardial and pleural gas once the diaphragm is closed. The ventral-most portion of the defect is the most challenging to suture due to the angle needed to reach the hernia adjacent to the sternum. As the instrument tips are brought ventrally, movement of the surgeon's hands may be impeded by the inner thigh or ventral body wall of the patient. Placing the instrument ports more laterally may reduce this problem, and resection of the falciform fat, if not already performed, may also improve access to the ventral most extent of the hernia. Ending the simple continuous pattern with the suture assist device just dorsal to the ventral most extent of the hernia and using barbed suture with traditional needle drivers to place a final cruciate suture ventrally can help secure closure of the hernia ring ventrally. The pericardial catheter is withdrawn once suturing of the hernia is complete and pericardial gas withdrawn. Port sites are closed routinely.

CHALLENGES

Because the PPDH allows communication between the peritoneal and pericardial cavities, insufflation of the abdomen can lead to pericardial insufflation and severe hypotension. In the author's experience, hypotension often occurs once herniated contents have been reduced. Initial insufflation pressures may be set at 5 to 8 mm Hg and blood pressure should be monitored very closely, particularly following reduction. If hypotension develops, insufflation may be decreased or temporarily stopped to allow blood pressure to normalize before resuming insufflation at 3 to 5 mm Hg to complete herniorrhaphy. Because of the location of diaphragmatic hernias under the costal arch,

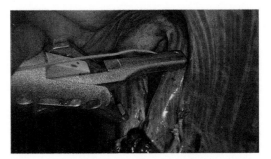

Fig. 5. Use of a suture assist device greatly facilitates closure of the diaphragmatic defect as the needle of the device is positioned parallel to the diaphragm to allow precise needle placement; this may reduce risk of tension pneumothorax compared to passing a traditional curved needle along the diaphragmatic defect.

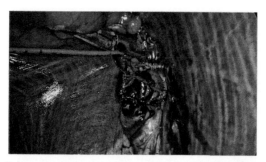

Fig. 6. The pericardial space is evacuated by passing a pericardiocentesis catheter through the herniorrhaphy prior to complete closure of the defect. Once the hernia is completely closed, insufflation is removed via the pericardial catheter and the catheter is withdrawn from the pericardial space.

the rigid thoracic wall can provide additional lift, reducing or eliminating the need for insufflation. Alternatively, herniorrhaphy may be performed using lift laparoscopy. In lieu of a designated device for lift laparoscopy, the author has placed a temporary percutaneous suture around the xiphoid cartilage using heavy gauge suture for an assistant to hold while the surgeon finishes herniorrhaphy with minimal insufflation. A novel device utilizing percutaneous sutures to facilitate gasless laparoscopic diaphragmatic herniorrhaphy was recently described.[10] This device, which includes a 3-dimensional–printed component to incorporate slots for hemostatic forceps, was evaluated for use in cadaveric diaphragmatic herniorrhaphy with intracorporeal suturing and mesh implantation and may be useful for laparoscopic herniorrhaphy in clinical cases (**Fig. 7**).

Although PPDH repair can usually be completed without entering the pleural space, accidental breach of the pleural space during laparoscopic repair can lead to hypoxemia and life-threatening tension pneumothorax. Oxygenation should be monitored carefully and the pleural spaced tapped if refractory hypoxemia develops. Some surgeons prefer to place a thoracoscopic cannula or thoracic drain at the beginning of the procedure to eliminate risk of a tension pneumothorax. In the author's experience, tension pneumothorax is most likely to occur when the needle is passed through the diaphragm during herniorrhaphy.

Preliminary data collected on laparoscopic PPDH herniorrhaphy performed in a small number of cats suggests high mortality in this species with laparoscopic repair. Of 3cats undergoing laparoscopic PPDH herniorrhaphy for which data has been retrospectively collected, 1 cat was converted to a laparotomy due to extensive adhesions and 2 suffered cardiopulmonary arrest during suturing of the diaphragm. The cause of death was unknown in both cats but suspected to be related to tension pneumothorax in 1 of the cats. It is possible that cats may be more susceptible to the effects of pericardial insufflation; their small size may also increase the risk of accidental penetration of the pleural space while suturing the diaphragm, potentially increasing the risk of tension pneumothorax. Until further research is performed to evaluate whether laparoscopic PPDH herniorrhaphy is safe in cats; the author recommends caution in considering this laparoscopic procedure in cats.

Rarely, the size of a PPDH may preclude primary repair via suturing of the hernia's edges. The use of mesh has been reported in the laparoscopic repair of a pleuroperitoneal hernia in a dog.[11] Mesh can be cut to match the size of the defect, inserted through a cannula, and sutured to the edges of the defect using simple interrupted intracorporeal sutures (**Fig. 8**).

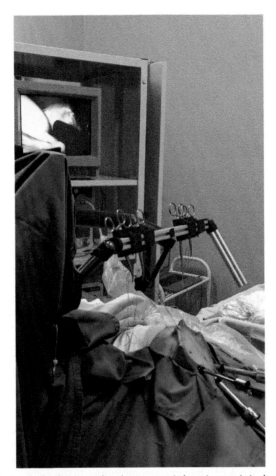

Fig. 7. A novel device to facilitate gasless laparoscopic hernia repair is shown. Percutaneous sutures are taken of the cranial abdominal wall and the associated hemostats are anchored to a frame to facilitate targeted lift laparoscopy. (*Photo courtesy of* Mauricio Brun.)

As mentioned previously, intrapericardial cysts may occur concurrently with PPDH. These cysts may be treated thoracoscopically.[7,12] If an intrapericardial cyst is detected on preoperative imaging, laparoscopic PPDH herniorrhaphy may be combined with thoracoscopic intrapericardial cyst resection. Once the hernia is repaired, any insufflation is stopped and thoracoscopic ports placed to resect the intrapericardial cyst. In the author's limited experience, the dorsal location of the cyst in close association with the caudal vena cava prevented resection within the pericardium via laparoscopy and pericardioscopy. It is possible that a more ventrally located cyst could be resected through a laparoscopic approach prior to hernia repair if the patient tolerates sustained pneumopericardium.

POSTOPERATIVE CARE AND OUTCOME

Postoperative recovery from laparoscopic PPDH herniorrhaphy is similar to that for other laparoscopic procedures. The displacement or compression of pulmonary

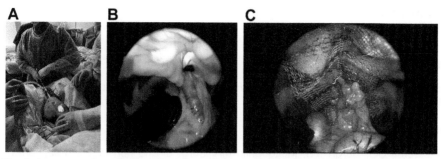

Fig. 8. Intraoperative photos of a minimally invasive repair of a substernal hernia and peritoneal-pericardial diaphragmatic hernia (PPDH). (*A*) shows the substernal defect. (*B*) shows the laparoscopic view of the contiguous substernal and peritoneal-pericardial hernias prior to reduction. (*C*) shows the laparoscopic view of the combined hernia repairs with mesh implantation. Omentum is draped over the cranial aspect of the mesh at the site of the PPDH herniorrhaphy. (Photos courtesy of Alex Chernov.)

tissue with PPDH is generally limited enough that concern for re-expansion pulmonary edema is not warranted. If a thoracostomy drain is placed for pleural drainage intraoperatively, the drain can usually be removed within 8 to 24 hours postoperatively if small or negligible volumes of fluid and air are obtained. Systemic blood pressure should be checked during recovery to ensure that there is no residual hypotension from pericardial insufflation.

Thoracic radiographs taken 2 years after laparoscopic PPDH repair in 1 dog were suggestive of re-herniation of adipose tissue into the pericardial space. For this reason, postoperative radiographs taken immediately postoperatively may be helpful as a basis for comparison should failure of the herniorrhaphy be suspected in the future.

SUMMARY

In summary, laparoscopic PPDH repair is a feasible minimally invasive option for dogs with PPDH. More evidence is needed before recommending this procedure in cats. Careful case selection and patient monitoring are critical for successful laparoscopic herniorrhaphy. Substantial liver herniation and/or the presence of extensive adhesions may require conversion to open celiotomy. Tension pneumothorax and severe systemic hypotension are potential life-threatening intraoperative risks that can be quickly addressed with careful monitoring.

CLINICS CARE POINTS

- Lift or "gasless" laparoscopy may be useful to avoid effects of pericardial insufflation.
- Initial abdominal insufflation should not exceed 8 mm Hg and may need to be decreased to 3 to 5 mm Hg (or temporarily stopped) once the hernia is reduced or earlier if the patient is showing signs of refractory hypotension.
- Tension pneumothorax may occur when dissecting adhesions or suturing the diaphragm; rapid evacuation of the pleural space via thoracoscopic cannula or thoracic drain may be indicated.
- Steep reverse Trendelenburg positioning can assist in reducing herniated organs.
- A suture assist device greatly facilitates closure of the diaphragmatic defect.

DISCLOSURE

The author has nothing to disclose.

SUPPLEMENTARY DATA

Supplementary data related to this article can be found online at https://doi.org/10.1016/j.cvsm.2024.02.003.

REFERENCES

1. Burns CG, Bergh MS, McLoughlin MA. Surgical and nonsurgical treatment of peritoneopericardial diaphragmatic hernia in dogs and cats: 58 cases (1999–2008). J Am Vet Med Assoc 2013;242(5):643–50.
2. Evans SM, Biery DN. Congenital peritoneopericardial diaphragmatic hernia in the dog and cat: a literature review and 17 additional case histories. Vet Radiol 1980;21(3):108–16.
3. Banz AC, Gottfried SD. Peritoneopericardial diaphragmatic hernia: a retrospective study of 31 cats and eight dogs. J Am Anim Hosp Assoc 2010;46(6):398–404.
4. Morgan KR, Singh A, Giuffrida MA, et al. Outcome after surgical and conservative treatments of canine peritoneopericardial diaphragmatic hernia: A multi-institutional study of 128 dogs. Vet Surg 2020;49(1):138–45.
5. Smolec O, Vnuk D, Brkljača Bottegaro N, et al. Repair of recurrent peritoneopericardial hernia in a dog, using polypropylene mesh and an autologous pericardial flap. Vet Arh 2018;88(3):427–35.
6. Reimer SB, Kyles AE, Filipowicz DE, et al. Long-term outcome of cats treated conservatively or surgically for peritoneopericardial diaphragmatic hernia: 66 cases (1987–2002). J Am Vet Med Assoc 2004;224(5):728–32.
7. Scharf VF, Iannettoni M, Anciano C. Laparoscopic peritoneopericardial herniorrhaphy in 2 dogs. Can Vet J 2021;63(9):947–52.
8. Sisson D, Thomas WP, Reed J, et al. Intrapericardial cysts in the dog. J Vet Intern Med 1993;7:364–9.
9. Raleigh JS, Mayhew PD, Visser LC, et al. The development of ventricular fibrillation as a complication of pericardiectomy in 16 dogs. Vet Surg 2022;51(4):611–9.
10. Brun MV, Sánchez-Margallo JA, Machado-Silva MA, et al. Use of a new device for gasless endosurgery in a laparoscopic diaphragmatic hernia repair ex vivo canine model: a pre-clinical study. Vet Med Sci 2022;8(2):460–8.
11. Hartmann HF, Basso PC, Faria KL, et al. Laparoscopic repair of congenital pleuroperitoneal hernia using a polypropylene mesh in a dog. Arq Bras Med Vet Zootec 2015;67(6):1547–53.
12. Chen CY, Fransson BA, Nylund AM. Intrapericardial cystic hematoma in a dog treated by thoracoscopic subtotal pericardectomy. J Am Vet Med Assoc 2017;250(8):894–9.

Augmenting Laparoscopic Surgery with Fluorescence Imaging

Chris Thomson, DVM

KEYWORDS

- Near-infrared • Fluorescence-guided surgery • Laparoscopy
- Minimally invasive surgery

KEY POINTS

- Near-infrared fluorescence imaging allows for live, intraoperative contrast enhancement of various systems (vascular, lymphatic, and urinary) for improved tissue identification.
- Future directions within veterinary laparoscopy should be targeted toward optimization and standardization of dosing, intraoperative perfusion imaging, and the use of cancer-specific probes.
- Indocyanine green is the most commonly employed near-infrared agent, due to it's safety, ease of use, and commercial availability.

BACKGROUND

Fluorescence is defined as the ability of a compound to absorb light at one wavelength and emit that light energy at a longer wavelength.[1] Fluorescence-guided surgery is performed through the use of target "probes" or fluorophores to highlight specific anatomy or molecular changes. Fluorescence-guided surgery can be used for open conventional surgery, but it is particularly easily applied to laparoscopic or thoracoscopic surgery as the procedures are being performed through a telescope in which light filters can be applied, a digital camera, and video screen. Given the high cross-over between open surgery and laparoscopic surgery uses, this narrative review will discuss both uses of the technology.

Near-infrared fluorescence (NIRF) specifically uses the NIR spectrum of wavelength at 650 to 900 nm. The use of NIRF for surgery is becoming popular, due to the high signal-to-noise ratio (improved conspicuity of the image and decreased granularity), the high sensitivity of the technology (a small concentration of fluorophore is easily detected), and the widespread commercial availability of the equipment and inputs. NIRF also has the advantage of high light penetration due to lower absorption of water

Surgical Oncology, Veterinary Specialty Hospital - North County, by Ethos Veterinary Health, 2055 Montiel Road #104, San Marcos, CA 92069, USA
E-mail address: cthomson@ethosvet.com

Vet Clin Small Anim 54 (2024) 671–683
https://doi.org/10.1016/j.cvsm.2024.02.004
0195-5616/24/© 2024 Elsevier Inc. All rights reserved.

and oxy/deoxyhemoglobin. Depending on the tissue type and sensitivity of the device used, NIRF agents can be detected as far as 10 to 40 mm beneath tissue surfaces.[2]

EQUIPMENT AND INSTRUMENTATION

NIRF endoscopy combines a standard endoscope with white light capabilities with the fluorescence filters applied alongside a visual processor for producing high-definition fluorescent images. This can be done through paired image capture and image registration, or, more commonly, through a beam splitter and exchangeable NIR filters, in which the same field of view is used for both white light and NIRF. For many systems, the image can be switched from white light to various fluorescence modes at the click of a button or foot pedal, including an ability to overlay the fluorescent captured image with standard white light imaging. Standard light sources can be used (halogen, xenon, light-emitting diode, or diode laser). The endoscopes use infrared light at wavelengths greater than 800 nm, along with, or separate from, normal visible white light at wavelengths around 760 nm.

Several commercially available NIRF endoscopes have been used clinically, including the Storz IMAGE1 S Rubina (Karl Storz, Tuttlingen, Germany), Arthrex SynergyID (Arthrex, Naples, FL), Wolf ENDOCAM Logic (Richard Wolf Medical Systems, Vernon Hills, IL), and Amnotec VEQTRON (AMNOTEC International Medical, Neuhausen ob Eck, Germany) systems. Additionally, there are several open field NIRF imaging devices, including Pulsion Medical IC-View, Mizuho HyperEye (Mizho Medical Corporation, Tokyo, Japan), Stryker SPY-PHI (Stryker, Portage, MI), Hamamatsu Photonics PDE-Neo II (Hamamatsu, Hamamatsu-City, Japan), Intuitive Surgical's Firefly system (Intuitive Surgical, Sunnyvale, CA), Karl Storz VitomII (Karl Storz, Tuttlingen, Germany), and many others.

INDOCYANINE GREEN

The most commonly used NIRF fluorophore in clinical practice is indocyanine green (ICG). ICG was developed for NIR photography in 1955 by Kodak Research Laboratories and was approved by the US Food and Drug Administration for clinical use in 1956. It is a water-soluble compound that emits fluorescence when stimulated either by an NIR light or by a laser beam. The peak fluorescence wavelength is 800 to 840 nm in water or tissue. ICG immediately binds to plasma proteins, is rapidly processed by the liver, and is excreted in bile. The plasma half-life is only 6 to 19 minutes in dogs.[3] The short half-life allows for repeated applications when necessary. However, pneumoperitoneum induces a decrease in splanchnic blood flow, including to the liver and kidneys, which increases the ICG half-life and reduces the ICG clearance in the splanchnic organs by 32%.[4]

ICG works well within lymphatics due to the protein binding of the compound paired with the high protein content in the lymph. ICG preferentially binds to alpha-1 lipoprotein, particularly high-density lipoproteins, more so than albumin.[5]

ICG most commonly comes as a powder stored in vials, which is diluted tableside with sterile water, at various concentrations and administered to the patient. According to the package insert, the compound is unstable in an aqueous solution and is recommended to be used within 6 hours. Under experimental conditions, when diluted in water and stored at 4°C in the dark, ICG was stable and only lost 20% of its fluorescence intensity over 3 days.[6] The powdered vital dye is soluble in sterile water but is not readily soluble in saline. Therefore, if an isotonic solution is desired, ICG should first be dissolved in water and subsequently diluted with saline.[5] There are ongoing veterinary studies evaluating the efficacy of ICG in various storage conditions and lengths of time, which will potentially aid in the prolonged use of a single 25 mg vial.

ICG has been reported as associated with minimal to no risk of adverse effects at standard doses, with no reported phototoxicity, high safety profile (median lethal dose [LD_{50}] of 50–80 mg/kg for rodents),[7] and only rare anaphylaxis case reports being described.[8] Other suggested adverse reactions include injection site or skin irritation, eye contact irritation, respiratory irritation on inhalation, nausea, fever, and anaphylactic shock.

Importantly, for clinical use, intravenously administered ICG can cause transient misreadings of pulse oximetry due to the interference with the plasma light absorption in the optical spectral monitors. In humans, this has been found to be mild (1.6%–4% decrease), dose dependent, and short lived (nadir at 57 seconds, time to recover 3.6 minutes).[9]

An interesting phenomenon of ICG NIRF is the quenching effect. This is defined as a lack of linear relationship between the dose of ICG administered and the fluorescence intensity. The intensity initially increases with increasing concentration, peaks, then decreases at subsequently higher concentrations (ie, higher doses result in less intense fluorescence). While this is not fully understood, it is thought to be due to effects of "excited-state reactions, energy transfer, and formational collisions" that cause the ICG molecules to self-absorb the fluorescence photos.[10]

Doses reported in veterinary medicine have ranged from 0.02 mg/kg[11] (lymphatic study) to 5 mg/kg[12] (using delayed phenomenon for tumor detection). Most lymphatic studies are on the lowest end of the dosing spectrum (0.01–0.1 mg/kg peritumorally); angiographic studies are often dosed less on patient size and more on a bolus injection (2.5 mg per patient *not* per kg or 1 mL of 2.5 mg/mL solution intravenously); and the second window dosing is often the highest, with doses around 3 to 5 mg/kg administered intravenously roughly 24 hours prior to surgery.

INDICATIONS

The use of ICG NIRF was originally described for evaluating cardiac output, hepatic function, and ophthalmic angiography. Following intradermal, submucosal, or subcutaneous injection, the ICG is dispersed in the lipoproteins, drawn to lymphatics, and subsequently gathered in lymph nodes. This allows for lymphangiography studies of lymphatic vessels (including the thoracic duct and cisterna chyli) and lymph nodes (including sentinel lymph nodes [SLNs]). When administered intravenously, the ICG is similarly bound to plasma proteins that allows for maintenance in the vascular system. This allows for studies of the vascular supply, tissue perfusion, and clearance. Given that ICG is excreted by the liver, it accumulates in liver tissue and ultimately in the bile. This allows for visualization of the biliary system for fluorescent cholangiography. Lastly, the ICG can be directly injected into other lumens (airway, ureters, and bowel) for intraoperative localization and leak testing. As previously discussed, ICG is generally considered nontoxic, unless there is a known iodine allergy.[13]

ANGIOGRAPHY

Given the protein-bound nature with a fast serum half-life of ICG, it is a valuable option to be used for intraoperative angiography. The fluorescent angiogram can be used to evaluate the arterial supply, tissue perfusion, uptake, distribution, and subsequent clearance and venous vasculature. And given the clearance of the dye and high safety profile of the compound, intraoperative angiograms can be repeated.

Tissue perfusion is an important assessment for many surgeries and surgical diseases, particularly for the bowel. ICG NIRF has been utilized for perfusion assessment of the large and small intestines in humans undergoing resection and anastomosis. Following NIR angiography in patients undergoing bowel resection and anastamosis, the surgical plan was altered in 5.6% of patients, due to adjusted assessment of tissue perfusion.[14] Additionally, in a prospective trial, the incidence of anastomotic leakage was reduced from 9% in the control group to 5% in cases in which an ICG NIR angiogram was performed for laparoscopic colorectal surgery.[15]

In veterinary medicine, little is reported on the indication, feasibility, and use of ICG NIRF for gastrointestinal perfusion studies. One abstract[16] has reported the use of ICG angiography to assess gastric perfusion and guide resection associated with gastric dilatation and volvulus in dogs. The authors describe ICG angiography via 0.15 mg/kg intravenous (IV) following gastric derotation, which prompted resection and guided margins for a partial gastrectomy in 2 out of 8 patients. While found to be safe and feasible in this setting, the accuracy and predictive value of ICG NIRF for gastrointestinal ischemia in veterinary medicine warrants additional study. When performed in humans, there is controversy as to what indicates true ischemia, as some authors describe the use of a "90 seconds rule," in which perfusion is only considered true if it appears within the first 90 seconds of initial tissue enhancement.

One area of interest for the use of NIR angiography is for the evaluation of the vascular supply for adrenal tumors. ICG has been used intraoperatively for radical adrenalectomy in people to aid in identifying the gland, guiding dissection, and even sparing normal adrenal tissue.[17–19] Data on ICG NIRF surgery for robotic and laparoscopic adrenalectomy in people suggest that its use can differentiate tumor type,[20] improve the speed of surgery, quality of dissection, reduce bleeding, and capsular violation.[21] Laparoscopic adrenalectomy is associated with excellent outcomes in veterinary medicine, particularly when performed from experienced centers.[22] While NIRF laparoscopic adrenalectomy has yet to be reported on in veterinary medicine, the author and several others are actively performing studies on ICG NIRF for adrenal surgery in dogs and cats. This may be of particular importance for patients with bilateral disease, if the technique ultimately allows for differentiation of malignancy and tumor type in veterinary patients. **Fig. 1** describes the use of NIRF for a dog with an adrenal tumor.

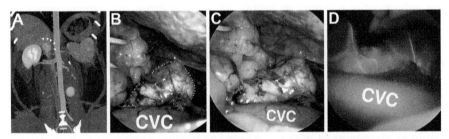

Fig. 1. Adrenal. (*A*) Coronal view of a postcontrast CT scan of the abdomen in a dog with a right-sided adrenal tumor, which is identified with the arrowheads. (*B*) White light image of the right sided adrenal tumor, identified with a dotted white line. The caudal vena cava (CVC) can be seen coursing at the bottom of the screen; cranial is to the right of the image. The liver can be seen across the top of the image and the cranial pole of the right kidney can be observed being retracted on the left side of the image. (*C*) ICG NIRF angiogram of the adrenal tumor with a green overlay. The angiogram is currently in an arterial phase, as demonstrated by the bright green arteries identified going to the adrenal tumor cranially and caudally. (*D*) Similar image to (*C*) (ICG NIRF angiogram in arterial phase) but with the monochromatic view (no white light turned on, just the NIRF filter with a monochromatic display).

While not associated with laparoscopy, NIRF angiography has been used in veterinary medicine for assisting in the identification of arterial vascular supply to cutaneous axial pattern flaps (APF). This has been reported for the superficial brachial APF in dogs[23] and the caudal auricular APF in cats.[24] **Fig. 2** demonstrates ICG NIRF of a deep circumflex iliac APF. Intraoperative angiogram was performed with ICG and an exoscope, confirming the location of the artery deep within the fatty tissue. NIRF angiograms for APFs have the potential to improve the planning and execution of raising the flaps to minimize acute ischemia related to individual vascular anatomy.

LYMPHANGIOGRAPHY

Following submucosal, subcutaneous, or intradermal injection, ICG disperses in the lymphatics, allowing visualization of lymphatic vessels and lymph nodes. The SLN is the first draining node from a tumor. In surgical oncology, if the first draining node is considered negative for metastasis, others are often assumed to be negative as well. Different types of lymphatic tracers have been used, including radioisotopes and dyes (technetium-99m, various blue dyes [sulfan, indigo carmine, and isosulfan]). Given its tropism for lymphatic tissue from protein binding, and the low incidence of allergic reactions, ICG has been considered advantageous to other lymphatic tracers due to the depth of visualization, high accuracy of tissue perception, and ability to avoid risk of radiation exposure.[13] Several studies have compared the use of ICG, blue dyes, and radioisotope lymphography alone or in conjunction and, in general, have found that NIRF provides a higher detection rate and lower false-negative rate than other options.[25–27] In veterinary medicine, a prospective study comparing ICG NIRF lymphangiogram versus methylene blue has been performed for oral tumors and found that NIRF identified a greater proportion of SLN (91%) compared to methylene blue (50%).[28]

In humans, the ICG is commonly injected peritumorally, with doses ranging from 1.25 to 25 mg per person (*not* per kg). The ability to detect SLNs varies between

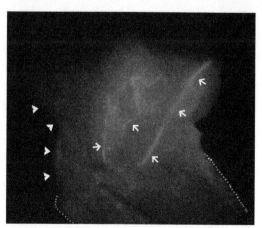

Fig. 2. APF angiography. Following the removal of a soft tissue sarcoma, this patient had primary closure with a deep circumflex iliac APF. Intraoperative angiogram was performed with ICG and an exoscope, confirming the location of the artery deep within the fatty tissue. The dotted line represents the donor bed, the arrowheads are at one of the margins of the created flap, and the arrows demonstrate the arterial supply to the flap. Imaging was performed without white light overlay and the fluorescence demonstrated in monochromatic display.

72% and 99%, depending on the technique used and the associated tumor type. While ICG lymphangiography appears highly useful for identifying the SLN, it is important to note that ICG is not cancer specific in this manner and identifies any draining lymph node, not specifically cancer-positive lymph nodes. Additionally, some tumors may be prone to skip metastasis, in which the sentinel node is negative but a further, secondary node may be positive for metastasis. False negatives may also occur, in which the lymph node that takes up contrast is not the draining lymph node, but secondary lymph node, particularly if there is obstruction of the lymphatic vessels leading to the actual sentinel node.

ICG can also be used to help map the location and recognition of a lymph node during extirpation. This is particularly useful in regions or patients with high fat deposition, such as the sublumbar space and pelvic canal. Complete validation has yet to be performed, but many surgeons are now performing laparoscopic sublumbar lymph node extirpation. This can be augmented by ICG NIRF to help identify the location of the lymph nodes within the retroperitoneal and pelvic adipose tissue. A cadaveric study in dogs identified that both intradermal and popliteal lymph node injection allowed for staining of the iliosacral lymph center.[29] In this study, a dose of 0.05 mg/kg was used, and the medial iliac lymph nodes were visualized to be fluorescent within 3 to 10 minutes following injection.

Fig. 3 describes the use of ICG NIRF for sublumbar lymphadenectomy for a dog with anal sac adenocarcinoma. The author now commonly performs sublumbar (iliac, hypogastric, and sacral) lymph node extirpation with laparoscopy, and the use of NIRF ICG allows efficient determination of node location. The ICG is typically dosed around 0.05 and 0.1 mg/kg diluted with sterile water for an injectate concentration that varies between 0.25 and 2.5 mg/mL, depending on the size of the patient. The ICG is administered subcutaneously in the region of the current or previous anal sac tumor, following port placement but prior to retroperitoneal reflection to minimize

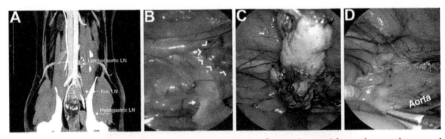

Fig. 3. Sublumbar lymph nodes. Laparoscopic view of a patient with anal sac adenocarcinoma metastasis to sublumbar lymph nodes. ICG was injected in the perineum prior to surgery, allowing for intraoperative lymphangiogram with the lymphatic vessel and SLN demonstrating profound fluorescence on the dorsal body wall. Imaging was performed with green overlay of fluorescence. (A) Postcontrast CT scan in a coronal view with a maximal intensity projection with a 13.3 mm thick slab. On all the laparoscopic images, cranial is to the left of the image and left lateral is to the top of the image. The arrowheads are around the lumbar aortic lymph node (LN), and there are arrows pointing to both the iliac lymph node and hypogastric lymph node on the left. Both of these lymph nodes are also outlined in a white dotted line. (B) The arrowheads are indicating the mildly fluorescent lymph node and the arrows indicate the fluorescent lymphatic vessel leading to the left external iliac LN. (C) Fluorescent LN after extirpation but before being retrieved from the body. (D) Fluorescent lymph node (left lumbar aortic LN) that was normal in size on the CT scan but due to the fluorescence, was extirpated, and found to be metastatic. The aorta is labeled immediately axial to the node and the asterisk signifies the deep circumflex artery.

disruption of any lymphatic vessels. While the technique has been used with success for identifying the iliac, hypogastric, and even deep sacral lymph nodes during laparoscopic extirpation, this technique has yet to be validated for identifying the true SLN. However, from this technique, additional lymph nodes that were found to be of normal size on preoperative computed tomography (CT) but fluorescent intraoperatively have been extirpated and found to be positive for metastasis, including a small accessory (lumbar aortic) lymph node near the deep circumflex artery (see **Fig.** 3D), and a colonic lymph node (**Fig. 4**).

CHOLANGIOGRAPHY

Due to the hepatic clearance and biliary excretion, ICG is a valuable fluorophore for imaging of the liver and biliary system following an IV injection. In dogs, the excretion into the bile is relatively quick, with 97% of ICG excreted unchanged within 6 hours of an intravenous injection.[30] The use of ICG NIRF for laparoscopic cholecystectomy in people is now commonplace for intraoperative cholangiograms. A prospective observational study comparing standard white light versus NIRF cholangiography was performed at 29 human surgical centers to evaluate whether NIRF would improve the visualization of the "critical view of safety" during laparoscopic cholecystectomy performed by surgical trainees. They found that the use of NIRF allowed for higher rates of visualization of the critical view of safety with no added operative time and a lower surgical workload.[31] Additionally, the use of NIRF cholangiography during laparoscopic cholecystectomies in humans decreased the rate of conversion to open surgery, decreased the incidence of bile duct injuries, and had an overall shorter operative time.[32]

A valuable study has been recently published[33] in veterinary medicine in which 2 doses of ICG administered at 2 time points prior to cholangiography was performed in dogs. The goal of the study was to optimize the dose and timing of ICG administration for optimal imaging of the biliary tree. They found that ICG could be visualized within 20 minutes and peaked at 100 minutes. Both low (0.05 mg/kg) and high (0.25 mg/kg) dose injections resulted in cystic duct fluorescence, with the low dose achieving better contrast between the biliary tree and the liver. The contrast ratio (cystic duct and background liver) was better to visualize the cystic duct at the later time course (around 300 minutes after injection). This study suggests that a lower dose (0.05 mg/kg) given 3 to 5 hours prior to expected surgical timing may provide the best visualization of the cystic duct during laparoscopic cholecystectomy.

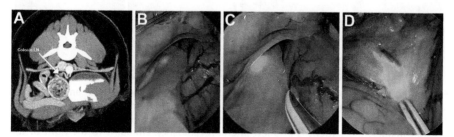

Fig. 4. Colonic lymph node. In the same patient as **Fig. 3**, on fluorescent laparoscopic exploration, it was found that there was a highly fluorescent colonic LN. (*A*) Postcontrast, axial view of the patient with the small colonic lymph node identified with an arrow. (*B* and *C*) Marked fluorescence of the lymph node within the colonic mesentery; the colon can be observed to the right of the images. (*D*) Fluorescent lymph node along with the fluorescent lymphatic vessels leading to the LN. This lymph node was extirpated and found to have metastatic anal sac adenocarcinoma cells within it.

DELAYED PHENOMENON AND NEOPLASTIC DIFFERENTIATION

A unique feature of ICG NIRF is the enhanced permeability and retention effect within tumors. This is described as a passive accumulation of the ICG fluorophore in the neoplastic tissues, allowing intraoperative differentiation between neoplastic tissues and normal tissues. The technique is not completely accurate for neoplasia only, due to the retention of ICG within inflammatory tissue as well. However, the use of ICG NIRF can still be beneficial during open and endoscopic surgery for an increased detection of neoplastic tissue and margin assessment.

The reports of ICG NIRF for second window evaluation of neoplasia in veterinary medicine are currently limited. Its use in humans is common for liver tumors,[34,35] pancreatic tumors,[36,37] renal cancer,[38] gastrointestinal cancers,[39] and urogenital tumors.[40]

A prospective[41] and subsequently validated[42] approach was performed in kidney tumors, in which an initial low dosage of ICG is administered (1.25 mg IV per person) as a test, followed by a second dose that was calibrated to the patient and tumor from the first dose. This allowed an optimized dose to differentiate the fluorescent pattern (neoplastic vs normal tissue) successfully in 87% of renal tumors, providing a low positive surgical margin rate (0.3%)[42] during partial nephrectomy. While most patients in veterinary medicine are undergoing a radical nephrectomy, the use of ICG still allows for an intraoperative assessment of vasculature, tumor identification, and has the potential to provide information on renal perfusion. **Fig. 5** provides an example of ICG used during a laparoscopic nephrectomy for a renal cell carcinoma. In this instance, the ICG NIRF was used as an intraoperative angiogram, similar to what was described for adrenal tumors, and not using the second window effect.

One area of active clinical research in human NIR surgery is the use of ICG for informing tumor risk based on the fluorescent pattern to aid in determining benign versus malignant nodules. Sakurai and colleagues[43] described the use of ICG for detection and margin assessment of 104 dogs with liver nodules. They found that the intensity and fluorescent pattern of liver nodules was not significantly associated with the histologic diagnosis. While the sensitivity of residual fluorescence for

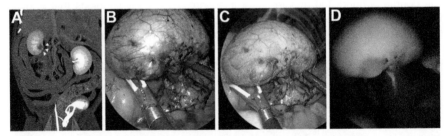

Fig. 5. Kidney. This image series describes a dog that was diagnosed with an incidentally identified renal cell carcinoma of the caudal pole of the right kidney. (*A*) Reformatted post-contrast, coronal view of a CT scan; the arrowheads point to the kidney tumor. For the laparoscopic images, the patient is in a left lateral recumbency, cranial is to the right of the image, right lateral is to the top of the images. (*B*) White light view of the right kidney following retroperitoneal dissection. The kidney is being elevated away from the CVC to best demonstrate the tumor and the renal hilus. (*C*) Same view but under a green overlay with an ICG NIRF angiogram, in a delayed/venous phase. (*D*) ICG NIRF angiogram in the parenchymal phase but with white light turned off and the NIRF under monochromatic mode. In this image, the renal tumor is clearly identified in the caudal pole and the renal vein can be identified within the perihilar fat.

incomplete resection was high (100%), only 3 out of 47 cases in which this was assessed were found to have incomplete margins. ICG has even been used as a tumor "tattoo" through the use of superselective transarterial embolization of the tertiary tumor feeding arteries with lipiodol to allow for improved intraoperative mass identification for endophytic renal tumors.[44]

Similar to renal tumors, the staining patterns of ICG for liver tumors has been well described in people. Given that ICG is processed by organic anion-transporting polypeptides (OATP) and sodium taurocholate cotransporting polypeptides (NTCP), the variable expression of these polypeptides in tumors allows for pattern recognition of their fluorescent pattern to an associated histology. As an example, in humans, well-differentiated hepatocellular carcinoma (HCCs) have a higher expression of OATP and NTCP that creates a high "total" fluorescent pattern in which the tumor is homogeneously fluorescent to the surrounding liver parenchyma.[45]

In veterinary medicine, this has been evaluated for dogs undergoing an open liver lobectomy in 2 retrospective studies. An initial case series of 12 dogs described the fluorescent patterns and started to evaluate the use of ICG NIRF for margin assessment.[46] In a follow-up study[43] from the same research group at Nihon University, they described the fluorescent imaging and margin assessment from 104 clinical

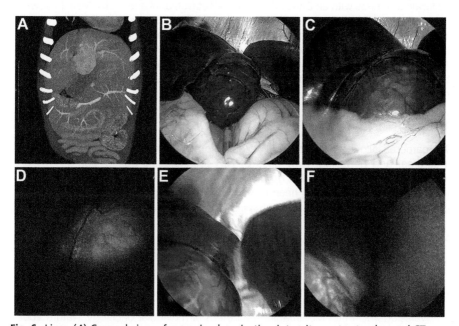

Fig. 6. Liver. (*A*) Coronal view of a maximal projection intensity contrast-enhanced CT scan of a patient with a hepatocellular carcinoma. The tumor can be found within the central division of the liver, immediately left lateral to the gallbladder. (*B*) Laparoscopic appearance of the liver tumor under white light endoscopy. (*C*) Correlated laparoscopic appearance of the liver tumor while utilizing a NIRF view under overlay settings with the Karl Storz Rubina endoscope. (*D*) Monochromatic view of the ICG NIRF image of the liver tumor. (*E*) Visualization of the liver tumor at the juncture of the quadrate lobe and left medial liver lobes, demonstrating the capsular deforming tumor. (*F*) Paired image of the quadrate lobe liver tumor that demonstrates fluorescence that extends proximally into the liver parenchyma, beyond the exophytic region of the liver tumor. This tissue was found to have residual neoplastic cells following an additional deep margin resection due to the residual fluorescence observed intraoperatively.

dog patients. The article describes 3 distinct fluorescent patterns (partial, whole, and ring hyperfluorescence) but found that the fluorescent intensity and pattern were not associated with the final histopathologic diagnosis. However, a subset of 47 dogs was evaluated for margin assessment. In these patients, they performed fluorescence imaging following tumor resection to evaluate if residual fluorescence in the wound bed was associated with an incomplete margin. By histology, only 3 out of 47 cases had incomplete margins; all 3 cases had positive residual fluorescence at the resection margin. Of the 44 cases with negative histologic margins, 34 out of 44 had no residual fluorescence in the wound bed; 10 out of 44 cases had positive residual fluorescence, associated with a false positive. This led to an incomplete margin residual fluorescence assessment sensitivity and specificity of 100% and 77.2%, respectively.

Fig. 6 describes a case of a laparoscopic liver lobectomy performed with the assistance of ICG NIRF. The patient was administered a 1.1 mg/kg dose of ICG roughly 24 hours prior to a CT scan and surgery. Surgery was performed through the combination of a single-incision multiport device (SILS, Medtronic, Inc. Minneapolis, MN) and an additional 5 mm port. The tumor was visualized in white light, NIRF overlay, and NIRF monochromatic and found to have evidence of fluorescence that extended roughly 2 cm beyond the capsular deforming mass. Surgery was performed to remove the lobulated mass with an Endo GIA stapler (Medtronic, Minneapolis, MN). Following tumor removal, it was observed that there was residual fluorescence along the proximal staple line, so an additional section of margins was excised via intraparenchymal dissection with a bipolar vessel-sealing device (Ligasure, Medtronic, Inc. Minneapolis, MN). The additional section of margins was found to have residual neoplastic cells at the staple line on final histopathology but was completely excised with the additional margins obtained.

SUMMARY

NIR cameras allow for real-time, high-definition visualization of vessels, anatomic structures, and perfusion. New uses of NIR technologies during laparoscopy are continuing to grow, for vascular, lymphatic, and oncologic-related techniques. Limitations exist, and future efforts need to be set for determining optimal dosing, tissue-specific fluorophores, and veterinary-specific techniques.

DISCLOSURE

The author has nothing to disclose.

REFERENCES

1. Weissleder R, Pittet MJ. Imaging in the era of molecular oncology. Nature 2008; 452(7187):580–9.
2. Unno N, Nishiyama M, Suzuki M, et al. Quantitative lymph imaging for assessment of lymph function using indocyanine green fluorescence lymphography. Eur J Vasc Endovasc Surg 2008;36(2):230–6.
3. Rakich PM, Prasse KW, Bjorling DE. Clearance of indocyanine green in dogs with partial hepatectomy, hepatic duct ligation, and passive hepatic congestion. Am J Vet Res 1987;48(9):1353–7.
4. Tuñón MJ, González P, Jorquera F, et al. Liver blood flow changes during laparoscopic surgery in pigs. A study of hepatic indocyanine green removal. Surg Endosc 1999;13(7):668–72.

5. Alander JT, Kaartinen I, Laakso A, et al. A review of indocyanine green fluorescent imaging in surgery. Int J Biomed Imaging 2012;2012:940585.

6. Mindt S, Karampinis I, John M, et al. Stability and degradation of indocyanine green in plasma, aqueous solution and whole blood. Photochem Photobiol Sci 2018;17(9):1189–96.

7. Green Indocyanine. Package insert. Drugs.com. Available at: https://www.drugs.com/pro/indocyanine-green.html. [Accessed 13 November 2023].

8. Frangioni JV. In vivo near-infrared fluorescence imaging. Curr Opin Chem Biol 2003;7(5):626–34.

9. Baek HY, Lee HJ, Kim JM, et al. Effects of intravenously administered indocyanine green on near-infrared cerebral oximetry and pulse oximetry readings. Korean J Anesthesiol 2015;68(2):122–7.

10. Using Raman spectroscopy to analyze Indocyanine Green (ICG) fluorescence. AZoM.com. 2022. Available at: https://www.azom.com/article.aspx?ArticleID=22137. [Accessed 12 December 2023].

11. Mitchell JW, Mayhew PD, Johnson EG, et al. Video-assisted thoracoscopic thoracic duct sealing is inconsistent when performed with a bipolar vessel-sealing device in healthy cats. Vet Surg 2018;47(S1):O84–90.

12. Holt D, Okusanya O, Judy R, et al. Intraoperative near-infrared imaging can distinguish cancer from normal tissue but not inflammation. PLoS One 2014; 9(7):e103342.

13. Dai ZY, Shen C, Mi XQ, et al. The primary application of indocyanine green fluorescence imaging in surgical oncology. Front Surg 2023;10:1077492.

14. Alius C, Tudor C, Badiu CD, et al. Indocyanine Green-Enhanced Colorectal Surgery-between Being Superfluous and Being a Game-Changer. Diagnostics 2020;10(10). https://doi.org/10.3390/diagnostics10100742.

15. De Nardi P, Elmore U, Maggi G, et al. Intraoperative angiography with indocyanine green to assess anastomosis perfusion in patients undergoing laparoscopic colorectal resection: results of a multicenter randomized controlled trial. Surg Endosc 2020;34(1):53–60.

16. Scientific Presentation Abstracts 2023 Veterinary Endoscopy Society Annual Conference July 6-8, Sorrento, Italy. Vet Surg 2023;O1–15.

17. Manny TB, Pompeo AS, Hemal AK. Robotic partial adrenalectomy using indocyanine green dye with near-infrared imaging: the initial clinical experience. Urology 2013;82(3):738–42.

18. Gokceimam M, Kahramangil B, Akbulut S, et al. Robotic Posterior Retroperitoneal Adrenalectomy: Patient Selection and Long-Term Outcomes. Ann Surg Oncol 2021;28(12):7497–505.

19. Colvin J, Zaidi N, Berber E. The utility of indocyanine green fluorescence imaging during robotic adrenalectomy. J Surg Oncol 2016;114(2):153–6.

20. Kahramangil B, Kose E, Berber E. Characterization of fluorescence patterns exhibited by different adrenal tumors: Determining the indications for indocyanine green use in adrenalectomy. Surgery 2018;164(5):972–7.

21. Aydin H, Donmez M, Kahramangil B, et al. A visual quantification of tissue distinction in robotic transabdominal lateral adrenalectomy: comparison of indocyanine green and conventional views. Surg Endosc 2022;36(1):607–13.

22. Mayhew PD, Massari F, Araya FL, et al. Laparoscopic adrenalectomy for resection of unilateral noninvasive adrenal masses in dogs is associated with excellent outcomes in experienced centers. J Am Vet Med Assoc 2023;261(12):1–8.

23. Michalik D, Nolff MC. Case Report: Indocyanine Green-Based Angiography for Real-Time Assessment of Superficial Brachialis Axial Pattern Flap Vascularization in Two Dogs. Front Vet Sci 2022;9:859875.

24. Quinlan ASF, Wainberg SH, Phillips E, et al. The use of near infrared fluorescence imaging with indocyanine green for vascular visualization in caudal auricular flaps in two cats. Vet Surg 2021;50(3):677–86.

25. Jung SY, Kim SK, Kim SW, et al. Comparison of sentinel lymph node biopsy guided by the multimodal method of indocyanine green fluorescence, radioisotope, and blue dye versus the radioisotope method in breast cancer: a randomized controlled trial. Ann Surg Oncol 2014;21(4):1254–9.

26. Hojo T, Nagao T, Kikuyama M, et al. Evaluation of sentinel node biopsy by combined fluorescent and dye method and lymph flow for breast cancer. Breast 2010; 19(3):210–3.

27. van der Vorst JR, Schaafsma BE, Verbeek FPR, et al. Randomized comparison of near-infrared fluorescence imaging using indocyanine green and 99(m) technetium with or without patent blue for the sentinel lymph node procedure in breast cancer patients. Ann Surg Oncol 2012;19(13):4104–11.

28. Wan J, Oblak ML, Ram A, et al. Determining agreement between preoperative computed tomography lymphography and indocyanine green near infrared fluorescence intraoperative imaging for sentinel lymph node mapping in dogs with oral tumours. Vet Comp Oncol 2021;19(2):295–303.

29. Sánchez-Margallo FM, Veloso Brun M, Sánchez-Margallo JA. Identification of intra-abdominal lymphatics in canine carcasses by laparoscopic fluorescence lymphography with intradermal and intrapopliteal ICG administration. PLoS One 2020;15(11):e0241992.

30. Ketterer SG, Wiegand BD, Rapaport E. Hepatic uptake and biliary excretion of indocyanine green and its use in estimation of hepatic blood flow in dogs. Am J Physiol 1960;199:481–4.

31. Ortenzi M, Corallino D, Botteri E, et al. Safety of laparoscopic cholecystectomy performed by trainee surgeons with different cholangiographic techniques (SCOTCH): a prospective non-randomized trial on the impact of fluorescent cholangiography during laparoscopic cholecystectomy performed by trainees. Surg Endosc 2023. https://doi.org/10.1007/s00464-023-10613-w.

32. Serban D, Badiu DC, Davitoiu D, et al. Systematic review of the role of indocyanine green near-infrared fluorescence in safe laparoscopic cholecystectomy (Review). Exp Ther Med 2022;23(2):187.

33. Larose PC, Brisson BA, Sanchez A, et al. Near-infrared fluorescence cholangiography in dogs: A pilot study. Vet Surg 2023. https://doi.org/10.1111/vsu.14007.

34. Ishizawa T, Masuda K, Urano Y, et al. Mechanistic background and clinical applications of indocyanine green fluorescence imaging of hepatocellular carcinoma. Ann Surg Oncol 2014;21(2):440–8.

35. Nakaseko Y, Ishizawa T, Saiura A. Fluorescence-guided surgery for liver tumors. J Surg Oncol 2018;118(2):324–31.

36. de Muynck LDAN, White KP, Alseidi A, et al. Consensus Statement on the Use of Near-Infrared Fluorescence Imaging during Pancreatic Cancer Surgery Based on a Delphi Study: Surgeons' Perspectives on Current Use and Future Recommendations. Cancers 2023;15(3). https://doi.org/10.3390/cancers15030652.

37. Li Z, Li Z, Ramos A, et al. Detection of pancreatic cancer by indocyanine green-assisted fluorescence imaging in the first and second near-infrared windows. Cancer Commun 2021;41(12):1431–4.

38. Feng J, Yang W, Qin H, et al. Clinical application of indocyanine green fluorescence imaging navigation for pediatric renal cancer. Front Pediatr 2023;11: 1108997.
39. Sposito C, Maspero M, Belotti P, et al. Indocyanine Green Fluorescence-Guided Surgery for Gastrointestinal Tumors: A Systematic Review. Ann Surg Open 2022; 3(3):e190.
40. Sheth RA, Upadhyay R, Stangenberg L, et al. Improved detection of ovarian cancer metastases by intraoperative quantitative fluorescence protease imaging in a pre-clinical model. Gynecol Oncol 2009;112(3):616–22.
41. Angell JE, Khemees TA, Abaza R. Optimization of near infrared fluorescence tumor localization during robotic partial nephrectomy. J Urol 2013;190(5):1668–73.
42. Sentell KT, Ferroni MC, Abaza R. Near-infrared fluorescence imaging for intraoperative margin assessment during robot-assisted partial nephrectomy. BJU Int 2020;126(2):259–64.
43. Sakurai N, Ishigaki K, Terai K, et al. Clinical impact of near-infrared fluorescence imaging with indocyanine green on surgical treatment for hepatic masses in dogs. BMC Vet Res 2022;18(1):374.
44. Nardis PG, Cipollari S, Lucatelli P, et al. Cone-Beam CT-Guided Transarterial Tagging of Endophytic Renal Tumors with Indocyanine Green for Robot-Assisted Partial Nephrectomy. J Vasc Interv Radiol 2022;33(8):934–41.
45. Potharazu AV, Gangemi A. Indocyanine green (ICG) fluorescence in robotic hepatobiliary surgery: A systematic review. Int J Med Robot 2023;19(1):e2485.
46. Iida G, Asano K, Seki M, et al. Intraoperative identification of canine hepatocellular carcinoma with indocyanine green fluorescent imaging. J Small Anim Pract 2013;54(11):594–600.

Near-infrared-guided Thoracoscopic Surgery and Future Near-infrared Targets

Chris Thomson, DVM*

KEYWORDS

- Near-infrared • Fluorescence-guided surgery • Thoracoscopy
- Minimally invasive surgery

KEY POINTS

- Use of indocyanine green (ICG) near-infrared fluorescence (NIRF) has been established and shows advantages over older dye agents such as methylene blue for thoracic duct visualization in small animals.
- ICG lymphangiography has been successful with both indirect and direct injections.
- Second window application of ICG NIRF may improve detection for lung tumors.
- Future clinical applications may include aerosolized ICG to detect pleural lesions, intraoperative sentinel lymph node mapping, and targeted NIRF probes.
- Clinical validation and guidelines are still lacking.

For many thoracic surgeries now, standard thoracotomies are being replaced by a less-invasive thoracoscopic or a thoracoscopic-assisted approach. While these techniques decrease pain, decrease morbidity, and, in some ways, improve the visualization of certain structures, it has inherent challenges. Challenges include positioning needs and a lack of bimanual digital palpation to identify small nodules or lymph nodes. Fluorescent imaging provides a unique opportunity to overcome some of these challenges and add to the visualization capacity of thoracoscopic surgery.

Fluorescence-guided surgery is performed through the use of target "probes" or fluorophores to highlight specific anatomy or molecular changes. More information on the mechanics and instrumentation regarding NIRF imaging can be found in the previous study in this book. To date, the use of near-infrared fluorescence (NIRF) imaging during thoracoscopy has mimicked that of laparoscopy, with its use in lymphatic studies, angiographic studies, and using the delayed phenomenon for tumor identification. Most NIRF used for thoracoscopy has similarly been performed with an

Surgical Oncology, Veterinary Specialty Hospital - North County, by Ethos Veterinary Health, 2055 Montiel Road. #104, San Marcos, CA 92069, USA
* 100 Main Street #502, Vista, CA 92084.
E-mail address: cthomson@ethosvet.com

Vet Clin Small Anim 54 (2024) 685–695
https://doi.org/10.1016/j.cvsm.2024.02.011
0195-5616/24/© 2024 Elsevier Inc. All rights reserved.

vetsmall.theclinics.com

extrinsic probe, indocyanine green (ICG). However, for lung tumors and metastatic lesions, additional effort is being pursued for other targeted extrinsic and intrinsic fluorophores, as will be discussed later in the article. While not exclusively veterinary data, this article intends to introduce the concept of fluorescent-guided thoracoscopic surgery and inspire further investigations on the contemporary and future use of this technology in veterinary medicine.

THORACIC LYMPHOGRAPHY

One of the most common and earliest clinical uses of NIRF in veterinary medicine was for thoracic duct (TD) identification.[1] The use of NIRF for TD lymphography is a perfect example of how the technology can improve intraoperative and postoperative outcomes. The use of NIRF for TD visualization allows for real-time identification of the multiple branches of the TD within the deeper layers of fat within the mediastinum. Interestingly, the clinical use of ICG NIRF TD lymphography in veterinary medicine helped to lead the way for its use in human intraoperative thoracoscopic NIRF lymphography[2–4]

Steffey and Mayhew[1] originally described the technique of NIRF lymphography for the TD for dogs with presumed idiopathic chylothorax. The technique was performed through the direct injection of ICG via 25 or 27 gauge needle into a lymph node (mesenteric via mini paracostal approach or popliteal through a small cutdown). NIRF of the TD was achieved in all 15 dogs. Dosage varied between 0.01 and 0.32 mg/kg (median 0.05 mg/kg), depending on the number of injections required for fluorescence. The time to fluorescence ranged from less than 1 minute to less than 25 minutes, largely depending on whether the fluorescence was achieved initially through the popliteal lymph node (LN) or if a mesenteric node approach was required.

General experiential recommendations from the authors of this study include placement of ports and initial pleural reflection performed prior to ICG injection, direct LN injection to allow for quick (<1–5 minutes) TD fluorescence, and recommended concentration of injectate is 0.25 to 0.5 mg/mL to not observe quenching of the TD. This study also confirmed the benefits observed with ICG NIRF lymphography, in that the NIRF lymphography identified the TD in all patients, often with additional observed branches, compared to methylene blue intraoperative lymphography which only correctly identified the TD in 44% (4 of 9 patients).

Follow up to this initial study includes several prospective and retrospective trials that have utilized a similar protocol for NIRF TD lymphography. A multi-institutional retrospective study of 39 dogs,[5] of which 24 had NIRF TD lymphography performed, found a long-term resolution of chylothorax in 91% of dogs that survived the perioperative period. A prospective single institutional study[6] of 26 dogs undergoing TD ligation, NIRF TD lymphography was performed and successful in 25 of 26 patients (96%), more so than methylene blue, in which only 2 of 6 patients (33%) had successful visualization of the TD.

The studies evaluating ICG NIRF lymphography for TD visualization use a combination of direct lymphography via popliteal node direct injection (following surgical cut down), mesenteric lymph node injection (ultrasound-guided injection or following mini paracostal surgical approach), or indirect lymphography via 4 quadrant perineal injection, mesenteric root injection, or intrametatarsal pad injection.[7] It has been suggested that indirect lymphography may not provide the same signal achieved with direct lymphography or speed of fluorescence. One study also reported on the use of a paracostal approach to the mesentery and the placement of a 26 gauge catheter directly into a mesenteric lymphatic duct for NIRF of the TD.[8] However, success of this technique was not reported.

Fig. 1 demonstrates a patient with idiopathic chylothorax that underwent a presurgical computed tomographic (CT) lymphogram, followed by TD ligation with the assistance of direct intraoperative ICG NIRF lymphography. In this case, a mesenteric lymph node was injected via ultrasound guidance with 1 mL of 2.5 mg/mL solution of ICG. Following injection, the TD was made visible and clipped with automatic endoscopic clips. Following the initial TD clipping, an additional lymphatic vessel, not previously observed on the thoracoscopic or CT lymphograms, became visible with the fluorescence and was subsequently clipped. This suggests that there may be "hidden/sleeper vessels" or nondistended lymphatic vessels that become distended with chylous fluid upon clipping of the main, higher flow thoracic lymphatic vessels. These situations demonstrate the immense value added from intraoperative NIRF lymphography to ensure complete obstruction of forward flow of the lymphatics during a TD ligation.

An alternative technique through the use of ultrasound-guided percutaneous injection in the liver has been evaluated.[9] In an experimental study using healthy Beagle dogs, the authors found that all patients (5 of 5) had NIRF visualization of the TD. They noted that the travel times were shorter than previously reported indirect lymphography studies, with an average time to fluorescence of 6 minutes. In this study, they used a 2.5 mg/mL solution of ICG, dosed at 0.1 mg/kg and diluted with sterile 0.9% NaCl to a total volume of 1 mL. As a technical consideration, the authors noted that in 3 of 5 cases, the injectate was found to be passing within the hepatic vasculature and required repositioning to allow for deposition into the liver parenchyma.

Little has been described for the use of NIRF lymphography for TD identification in cats, but the author and several others have used the technique successfully. A single

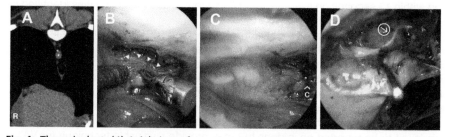

Fig. 1. Thoracic duct. (*A*) Axial view of a post-contrast CT lymphography scan of the thorax at the level of T10 in a dog with idiopathic chylothorax. In this image, the right is to the left of the screen, dorsal is to the top, the asterisk is labeling the aorta. Immediately adjacent to and dorsal to the aorta at this level was a single, right-sided thoracic duct. This correlated to the thoracic duct observed intraoperatively with the ICG NIRF lymphogram. (*B*) This is an intraoperative photo of the thoracic duct, as highlighted by the ICG lymphogram with the NIRF in a green overlay. A right-sided thoracoscopic approach was performed with 3 ports placed within the 8th to 10th intercostal spaces. The patient is positioned in a sternal recumbency; cranial is to the right of the image and dorsal is to the top of the images. The patient received 1 mL of a 2.5 mg/mL solution of ICG injected directly into a mesenteric lymph node under ultrasound guidance intraoperatively. The arrowheads indicate the presumed single thoracic duct, as it was being dissected free with the Maryland jaw dissector on the right hand of the image. (*C*) Intraoperative ICG NIRF lymphangiogram demonstrating ductal dilation of the caudal thoracic duct following placement of a single surgical clip on the thoracic duct. The clip is identified with the letter "C" and the arrowhead and the thoracic duct that was located caudal to this was found to have slowly dilated following clip placement. (*D*) New lymphatic vessel (identified with an *arrow* in a circle) that was observed dorsal and left lateral to the previously placed thoracic duct clips (seen lower in the image). This lymphatic vessel was not previously fluorescent prior to the placement of the clips, but following the pressure changes, became apparent and was subsequently clipped as well.

case series of 2 cats[10] described the use of perirectal injection for indirect TD lymphography for both a preoperative CT scan and for intraoperative TD detection. In this case series, a dose of ~4.5 mg/kg, diluted to 2.5 mg/mL was injected and allowed for detection of the fluorescence. While the time to fluorescence was not reported, it was noted that the TD was visible with NIRF for a full 15 minute observation period.

AEROSOLIZED INDOCYANINE GREEN

One unique opportunity for the use of ICG NIRF during thoracoscopic surgery is the use of aerosolized ICG. The use of aerosolized ICG has been documented in human thoracoscopic surgery to identify ground glass nodules, lung tumor margins, identification of the tracheobronchial tree within the mediastinum during esophagectomy,[11] and emphysematous lung disease. When performing aerosolized NIRF with ICG, patients are administered the reconstituted ICG in sterile water through a nebulizer system over 2 to 10 minutes.[11]

Applications of aerosolized ICG have yet to be published in veterinary medicine. However, using dogs as an experimental model, aerosolized ICG has been tested to identify emphysematous lung disease and for identification of pleural defects associated with postoperative air leaks.[12] To model a pleural defect, a 25 gauge needle was passed 2 mm into the pulmonary parenchyma and cauterized with electrosurgery at 30 W to create a pinhole-shaped defect. To identify the pleural defect and air leakage, a pediatric jet nebulizer was used to aerosolize 5 mL of 2.5 mg/mL ICG through an 8 French catheter located within the tracheal carina. The ICG was visualized within 13 seconds on average, up to 60 seconds, and the defect was identified in 24 of 25 instances (96%).

While this was a valuable evaluation of aerosolized ICG for pleural defects, the model represents defects/leaks that are created among normal appearing parenchyma. For clinical use, most areas of leakage are likely to be at a staple line or ligature line, where there is already exposed parenchyma at the site of the seal. As a follow-up study, the same group performed ICG leak testing in human patients undergoing video assisted thoracoscopic surgery (VATS) lung resection. They found the ICG leak test to have a higher detection rate than conventional sealing tests during thoracoscopy.[13] This is yet to be reported on in dogs but may provide a valuable technique for VATS lung lobe resection. Additionally, the technique provides a good reference for identifying pulmonary parenchymal changes at the pleural surface, suggesting the technique may have clinical use in veterinary patients diagnosed with pulmonary bulla or blebs.

NEAR-INFRARED FLUORESCENCE "SECOND WINDOW" FOR THORACOSCOPY

For small pulmonary nodules, several techniques have been attempted to improve localization and identification during thoracoscopic surgery. This includes the use of hook wires, direct injections of dyes (methylene blue), or simple anatomic and landmark-based resections derived from presurgical 3 dimensional imaging. However, these all have known complications, such as wire migration, pneumothorax, or leakage of methylene blue in the nearby areas. The use of ICG NIRF for small nodules within lungs has gained traction due to the ease of use, low toxicity, and minimal detrimental effects on the final histopathology.

Similar to what is observed in peripheral, musculoskeletal, and some visceral tumors, lung tumor fluorescence can be observed by the "second window" effect of ICG NIRF. This occurs when ICG is administered intravenously around 24 hours prior to the planned surgery. One of the initial studies that evaluated the second window phase for lung tumors was by Okusanya and colleagues.[14] In this trial, they administered ICG at 5 mg/kg intravenously 24 hours prior to surgery and had an 89% nodule detection rate (16 of 18) for target nodules identified on the preoperative CT scan. Additionally, they identified 5 nodules using ICG NIRF that were less than a centimeter in size; all of which were found to be metastatic nodules. This study was further supported by Mao and colleagues, in which they assessed for pulmonary nodules by standard white light, followed by ICG NIRF. The NIRF exploration identified an additional 9 nodules in 36 patients, for a total of 76 nodules identified and resected.

While ICG for the second window detection of pulmonary tumors has now been proven in multiple prospective studies, the specific dosing remains unknown. Most of the original articles on this topic used a standard 5 mg/kg injection intravenously, roughly 24 hours prior to surgery. This was based on an experimental mouse model in which 5 mg/kg was found to be optimal.[15] However, in a subsequent prospective "dose de-escalation" human study,[16] it was found that the optimal dose is dependent on the underlying histology. For patients with a primary lung tumor, the fluorescence activity (tumor-to-background ratio) was increased with increasing doses. However, for metastatic lesions, thymomas, or mesothelioma, a dose of 3 mg/kg was found to be optimal, as it both had the highest maximal fluorescence intensity of the tumor and simultaneously minimized the background fluorescence.

In veterinary medicine, the use of ICG for NIRF of lung tumors has been clinically reported in 40 dogs during open thoracotomy. The authors of this study used a dose of 2.0 mg/kg of ICG administered intravenously 12 to 24 hours prior to surgery. During surgery, a thoracotomy was performed to visualize the tumors and the lungs were visualized with a HyperEye infrared camera system (Mizuho Medical Co, Tokyo, Japan). The NIRF was feasible in all dogs, with every tumor identified to be fluorescent. Additionally, 2 fluorescent nodules were identified during NIRF imaging that were not identified preoperatively on the CT scan, one of which was a metastatic lesion and one of which was an inflammatory lesion of foamy macrophages. An attempt was made to evaluate whether NIRF could assist with intraoperative margin evaluation; however, the accuracy of this was only 60% when compared to histopathology as the gold standard. Additionally, the study evaluated for fluorescence and presence of metastasis in the tracheobronchial lymph nodes, and was found to have a sensitivity, specificity, and accuracy of 100%, 75%, and 85.7%, based on comparison to the lymph node histopathology in 7 dogs. Overall, this study suggests usefulness of ICG NIRF for lung tumor identification, a low diagnostic accuracy for margin assessment, but a high accuracy for detection of metastatic lymph nodes.

In contrast to IV injections of ICG prior to surgery, the use of intraoperative sentinel lymph node mapping through peritumoral injections has also been reported in humans.[17] When performed in this manner, 2.0 mL of 5 mg/mL ICG was injected around the tumor using a 25 gauge needle. Following injection, the injection sites were "closed" via surgical clips or pretied loop ligatures. The technique had an identification rate of 80% (25 of 31 patients). Subsequently, numerous prospective trials have reported on the use of ICG NIRF for sentinel lymph node mapping. Alterations to the technique include diluting the ICG in 20% human albumin, transpleural injections in aerated and nonaerated lungs, and transbronchial injection via a combined fluoroscopy and bronchoscopy platform (Illumisite platform, Medtronic, Minnesota, USA), with the latter reportedly to be preferred due to the extravasation observed in the transpleural approach.[18] While not yet published in veterinary medicine, this author is aware of preliminary discussions of transpleural injections for ICG NIRF sentinel lymph node mapping for lung tumors also in animal patients.

Another early evaluation of NIRF for lung tumors in veterinary medicine was performed by Keating and colleagues.[19] A folate receptor fluorophore (OTL0038) was utilized for tumor localization, lymph node sampling, and margin evaluation. They found that with the folate receptor fluorophore, all 10 dogs that underwent imaging and surgery were found to have successful fluorescence of their tumors. While not routinely performed, 3 abnormal lymph nodes were planned to be surgically excised due to their size, all found to be fluorescent, and all found to be positive for metastasis. This study used a folate-targeted contrast agent, folate-fluorescein isothiocyanate. Folate receptors have been found to be highly expressed in numerous cancer types so additional research using this fluorophore is warranted.

While yet to be published, the author has similarly used ICG NIRF for identification and resection of pulmonary metastasis in dogs during thoracoscopic metastasectomy. At a dose of 5 mg/kg or 25 mg/dog, whichever is less, administered 24 hours IV prior to surgery, metastatic pulmonary nodules have been observed clinically in dogs with tumors as small as 2 mm. For thoracoscopic metastasectomy, nodules may be small (<1 cm), not visible on the pleural surface, or hidden between segments of lobes. NIRF imaging for metastatic nodules has been shown to be valuable for this surgery and our Thomson CB, 2024, unpublished data will be available soon to further describe the technique.

Fig. 2 demonstrates a patient that underwent thoracoscopic metastasectomy. The patient developed 3 pulmonary nodules roughly 6 months following regional mammectomy for a high-grade mammary carcinoma. A preoperative CT scan identified the 3 nodules but 2 of the nodules were <5 mm in size. Intraoperative NIRF was used to aid in identification of these small nodules, which were poorly visible on routine white light thoracoscopic exploration. The 2 smaller nodules were easily identified via the second window NIRF and a monochromatic display. All 3 nodules were resected via thoracoscopy, the patient discharged within 18 hours after surgery. This patient is still alive over 6 months after the thoracoscopic metastasectomy.

CONTROVERSIES

As with the adoption of any new technology, there will be varied data on the ideal use. For NIRF, the optimal dosing, timing, and injection techniques, as well as the ideal equipment considerations are all still unknown. As the uses of NIRF continue to expand, it will be critical that the field develops techniques for validation and guidelines for use. There have been attempts at developing[20] and using[21,22] a staging system and assessment framework for fluorescence-guided surgery,[23] and it would be a good consideration for veterinary medicine to adopt a similar framework.

Much of NIRF in veterinary medicine is within the first or second stage of innovation development and evaluation,[20] namely the innovation stage in which new uses are in early reports, and the development phase in which the planned use of the technique is reported in small case series. It is vitally important during this phase that all technical modifications are reported in a detailed nature to allow an understanding on how these details may affect outcome. Similarly, there is a large learning curve of adopting the new technique, which should be clearly identified to avoid harm to patients. As we progress to the exploration and assessment stages, systematic data capture, development of research databases, and well-characterized and relevant outcome measures should be identified and agreed upon by key stakeholders in the field.

In addition to dosing considerations, a common controversy for evaluating NIRF is objective evaluation of the devices, the fluorophore, and fluorescence itself. To be able to optimize the dose or agent altogether, it is important to be able to first identify best

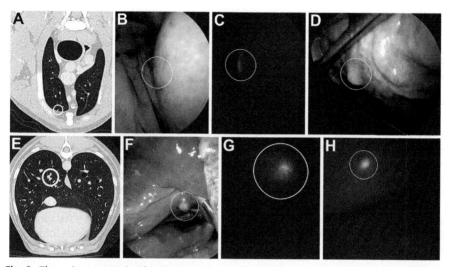

Fig. 2. Thoracic metastasis: This image series is of a patient that developed presumed pulmonary metastasis secondary to mammary carcinoma. (*A*) Axial slice of a preoperative CT scan; the patient's right is to the left of the image, dorsal is to the top of the image, the CT scan is in a lung optimized window. Toward the bottom/ventral aspect of the right cranial lung lobe was a solitary, ~2 mm pulmonary nodule as identified by the circle. (*B*) Intraoperative view under white light illumination. The patient is in a dorsal recumbency with the thoracoscope viewing the axial aspect of the right cranial lung lobe from a subxiphoid port. The pulmonary nodule is barely visible as a minimally capsular deforming nodule. (*C*) Mirrored image of (*B*) but with the white light turned off and a monochromatic NIRF window, which highlights the highly fluorescent nodule on the surface of the aerated lung. (*D*) Same pulmonary nodule with NIRF displayed as a green overlay while the nodule is being resected via a small partial lung lobectomy via pre-tied ligating suture loop. (*E*) Axial slice of the same CT scan but identifying the second, largest nodule within the right caudal lung lobe. (*F*) Axial view of the right caudal lung lobe following successful selective right caudal lung lobe bronchial blockade, with the nodule viewed with normal white light thoracoscopy. (*G*) Same nodule but displayed without white light and NIRF under monochromatic display. (*H*) A third, ~3 mm nodule within the right caudal lung lobe that was not visible on white light thoracoscopy but became visible under monochromatic NIRF view.

practices through objective testing. Currently, most research or clinical articles will evaluate fluorescence through a semi-quantification evaluation of the signal via maximal fluorescence intensity and tumor to background ratio of fluorescence. However, these values are highly dependent on various factors, including the distance of the camera to the subject, angulation of the camera, autofluorescence of tissues, and varied absorption or scatter of the fluorophore. Until a reproducible method has been validated, it is important for clinicians reporting on these techniques to best describe all variables that may be affecting the fluorescence interpretation.

FUTURE DEVELOPMENTS

Most intraoperative fluorescent imaging probes discussed here are extrinsic, that is, exogenous agents administered to patients, not "intrinsic" fluorescent agents such as collagen. Also, they are broad-spectrum agents that are not cancer specific but rely on properties of cancer tissue to allow for the fluorescence to occur. An opportunity exists to both alter the vehicle in which ICG is administered or to use an alternate fluorescent agent that is more tied to cancer-specific or disease-specific properties.

The vehicle in which ICG is administered has sparked recent research. This includes the use of nanoparticles or nanovectors that are used to slow elimination, evade immunosurveillance, or "functionalized" particles that carry ligands targeted to specific cell receptors.[24] Most of these compounds are still in an experimental, preapproval phase.

Compared to broad spectrum agents, targeted NIRF probes can take advantage of molecular-specific information that is targeted to cancer-specific cell receptors or antibodies. While a discussion on all of the active research on targeted probes is outside the scope of this narrative review, it is the hope that an introduction may stimulate further research and energy investment in veterinary medicine. Current research on targeted NIRF probes is ongoing for many cancer-specific cell receptors, such as folic acid, epidermal growth factor, carcinoembryonic antigen, fibroblast activation protein, y-glutamyl transpeptidase (GGT), somatostatin receptors, and vasoactive intestinal peptide.

In people 5 aminominolevulinic acid (5-ALA) has been used for various cancer-related applications. This includes lung tumors, high-grade gliomas,[25] melanoma,[26] and breast cancer.[27] 5-ALA is not directly a fluorophore or cancer cell receptor specific, but an amino acid and a precursor of protoporphyrine IX, part of the metabolic pathway that creates heme. The use of 5-ALA causes an excessive accumulation of protoporphyrin IX in neoplastic tissues, more so than what is observed in normal tissue. An added advantage of using 5-ALA as a tumor marker is that it can simultaneously be used as a therapeutic photosensitizer for photodynamic treatment.[28]

In veterinary medicine, 5-ALA has been reported for use in malignant mesothelioma, lung tumors,[29] mammary tumors,[30] and brain tumors.[31] 5-ALA had initial clinical testing performed in companion dogs as a preclinical model for humans with non-small cell lung cancer. In this trial,[29] 12 dogs with presumed primary lung tumors were administered 5-ALA at a dose of 20 mg/kg 2 to 4 hours prior to surgery. Six of 7 primary lung tumors were fluorescent but the tumors displayed heterogenous fluorescence and the fluorescence observed was not closely associated with margin status. However, only 1 of 5 nonpulmonary tumors displayed a fluorescent signal.

Osaki and colleagues[32] described the use of 5-ALA to target fluorescent mesothelioma nodules, as similarly described earlier with ICG. The use of NIRF to guide mesothelioma biopsies has been reported to enhance the detection of malignant lesions

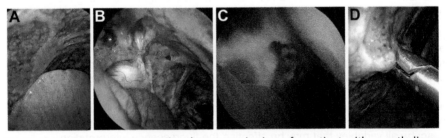

Fig. 3. Mesothelioma. Intraoperative thoracoscopic view of a patient with mesothelioma. The patient received a 1.5 mg/kg injection of ICG roughly 24 hours prior to surgery. (*A*) Normal white light appearance of the caudal pleural surface of the thoracic wall. (*B* and *C*) Paired images of the same anatomic view but displayed with standard white light (*B*) and monochromatic NIRF (*C*). During surgery, samples were collected from both fluorescent and nonfluorescent nodular regions. The regions of pathology that were fluorescent on NIRF were diagnosed as densely cellular mesothelioma, while the nodules that were nonfluorescent were diagnosed as collagenous fibrous proliferation. NIRF may allow for more directed targeting of neoplastic tissues during biopsy collection. (*D*) Biopsies being performed of the fluorescent regions of pleural pathology.

and avoid lesions that are more fibrotic or necrotic, potentially yielding a higher histologic detection rate. The author has similarly used NIRF for guidance of thoracoscopic biopsies for a dog with mesothelioma, demonstrated in **Fig. 3**. Interestingly, during the procedure, there were regions of highly fluorescent pathologic nodules, and nodules that contained little-to-no fluorescence. In a single patient evaluation, paired biopsies were performed of side-by-side, fluorescent and nonfluorescent pathologic areas. The regions of tissue that were biopsied in fluorescent nodules were diagnostic for densely cellular mesothelioma, while the regions of nonfluorescent yet still raised and pathologic tissue were diagnosed as regions of collagenous fibrous tissue.

SUMMARY

The use of near-infrared imaging during thoracoscopic surgery allows for not only circumventing many of the inherent problems that can be encountered by minimally invasive surgery, but may also open the door for improved visualization of pathologic tissue. Fluorescence-guided surgery can highlight specific anatomy or even molecular and neoplastic changes. More information on the mechanics and instrumentation regarding NIRF imaging can be found in the previous chapter in this book. To date, the use of NIRF imaging during thoracoscopy has mimicked that of laparoscopy, with its use in lymphatic studies, angiographic studies, and using the delayed phenomenon for tumor identification. Advancements in this field continue to be developed daily and the use of targeted probes will likely find a long-term place in thoracoscopic surgical oncology. Veterinary medicine has the chance to continue to be at the forefront with this technology and additional research should focus on further validating many of the techniques already in use.

CLINICS CARE POINTS

- Near infrared fluorescence imaging is a valuable tool that adds to the utility of thoracoscopy for thoracic surgery.
- NIRF lymphography aids in the identification of the thoracic ducts and provides real-time updates on lymphatic flow.
- Aerosolized ICG has yet to be fully explored in veterinary surgery but has the potential to aid in pulmonary parenchymal changes.
- Lung tumor fluorescence (primary or metastatic disease) provides a unique opportunity for improved visualization but futher work is needed on optimization of the technique.

DISCLOSURE

The author has nothing to disclose.

FUNDING

Part of the work described herein was funded by Ethos Discovery.

REFERENCES

1. Steffey MA, Mayhew PD. Use of direct near-infrared fluorescent lymphography for thoracoscopic thoracic duct identification in 15 dogs with chylothorax. Vet Surg 2018;47(2):267–76.

2. Yang F, Zhou J, Li H, et al. Near-infrared fluorescence-guided thoracoscopic surgical intervention for postoperative chylothorax. Interact Cardiovasc Thorac Surg 2018;26(2):171–5.

3. Londero F, Grossi W, Vecchiato M, et al. Fluorescence-Guided Identification of the Thoracic Duct by VATS for Treatment of Postoperative Chylothorax: A Short Case Series. Front Surg 2022;9:912351.

4. Shirotsuki R, Uchida H, Tanaka Y, et al. Novel thoracoscopic navigation surgery for neonatal chylothorax using indocyanine-green fluorescent lymphography. J Pediatr Surg 2018;53(6):1246–9.

5. Mayhew PD, Steffey MA, Fransson BA, et al. Long-term outcome of video-assisted thoracoscopic thoracic duct ligation and pericardectomy in dogs with chylothorax: A multi-institutional study of 39 cases. Vet Surg 2019;48(S1):O112–20.

6. Mayhew PD, Balsa IM, Stern JA, et al. Resolution, recurrence, and chyle redistribution after thoracic duct ligation with or without pericardiectomy in dogs with naturally occurring idiopathic chylothorax. J Am Vet Med Assoc 2022;261(5):696–704.

7. Scientific Presentation Abstracts 2019 Veterinary Endoscopy Society 16th Annual Scientific meeting, April 29-May 1, Lake Tahoe, CA. Vet Surg 2019;48(S2). https://doi.org/10.1111/vsu.13213.

8. Ishigaki K, Nagumo T, Sakurai N, et al. Triple-combination surgery with thoracic duct ligation, partial pericardiectomy, and cisterna chyli ablation for treatment of canine idiopathic chylothorax. J Vet Med Sci 2022;84(8):1079–83.

9. Korpita MF, Mayhew PD, Steffey MA, et al. Thoracoscopic detection of thoracic ducts after ultrasound-guided intrahepatic injection of indocyanine green detected by near-infrared fluorescence and methylene blue in dogs. Vet Surg 2022;51(Suppl 1):O118–27.

10. Kamijo K, Kanai E, Oishi M, et al. Perirectal injection of imaging materials for computed tomographic lymphography and near infrared fluorescent thoracoscopy in cats. Vet Med 2019;64(8):342–7.

11. Thammineedi SR, Patnaik SC, Nusrath S, et al. Evaluation of indocyanine green tracheobronchial fluorescence (ICG-TBF) via nebulization during minimally invasive esophagectomy. Dis Esophagus 2023. https://doi.org/10.1093/dote/doad059.

12. Yokota N, Go T, Fujiwara A, et al. A New Method for the Detection of Air Leaks Using Aerosolized Indocyanine Green. Ann Thorac Surg 2021;111(2):436–9.

13. Yokota N, Go T, Otsuki Y, et al. A New Method to Identify Air Leaks After Pulmonary Resection Using Indocyanine Green Aerosol. Ann Thorac Surg 2022;114(6):2067–72.

14. Okusanya OT, Holt D, Heitjan D, et al. Intraoperative near-infrared imaging can identify pulmonary nodules. Ann Thorac Surg 2014;98(4):1223–30.

15. Jiang JX, Keating JJ, Jesus EMD, et al. Optimization of the enhanced permeability and retention effect for near-infrared imaging of solid tumors with indocyanine green. Am J Nucl Med Mol Imaging 2015;5(4):390–400.

16. Newton AD, Predina JD, Corbett CJ, et al. Optimization of Second Window Indocyanine Green for Intraoperative Near-Infrared Imaging of Thoracic Malignancy. J Am Coll Surg 2019;228(2). https://doi.org/10.1016/j.jamcollsurg.2018.11.003.

17. Yamashita SI, Tokuishi K, Anami K, et al. Video-assisted thoracoscopic indocyanine green fluorescence imaging system shows sentinel lymph nodes in non-small-cell lung cancer. J Thorac Cardiovasc Surg 2011;141(1):141–4.

18. Stasiak F, Seitlinger J, Streit A, et al. Sentinel Lymph Node in Non-Small Cell Lung Cancer: Assessment of Feasibility and Safety by Near-Infrared Fluorescence

Imaging and Clinical Consequences. J Pers Med 2022;13(1). https://doi.org/10.3390/jpm13010090.

19. Keating JJ, Runge JJ, Singhal S, et al. Intraoperative near-infrared fluorescence imaging targeting folate receptors identifies lung cancer in a large-animal model. Cancer 2017;123(6):1051–60.

20. McCulloch P, Altman DG, Campbell WB, et al. No surgical innovation without evaluation: the IDEAL recommendations. Lancet 2009;374(9695):1105–12.

21. Ishizawa T, McCulloch P, Muehrcke D, et al. Assessing the development status of intraoperative fluorescence imaging for perfusion assessments, using the IDEAL framework. BMJ Surg Interv Health Technol 2021;3(1):e000088.

22. Esposito C, Del Conte F, Cerulo M, et al. Clinical application and technical standardization of indocyanine green (ICG) fluorescence imaging in pediatric minimally invasive surgery. Pediatr Surg Int 2019;35(10):1043–50.

23. Preziosi A, Paraboschi I, Giuliani S. Evaluating the Development Status of Fluorescence-Guided Surgery (FGS) in Pediatric Surgery Using the Idea, Development, Exploration, Assessment, and Long-Term Study (IDEAL) Framework. Children 2023;10(4). https://doi.org/10.3390/children10040689.

24. Egloff-Juras C, Bezdetnaya L, Dolivet G, et al. NIR fluorescence-guided tumor surgery: new strategies for the use of indocyanine green. Int J Nanomedicine 2019;14:7823–38.

25. Stummer W, Pichlmeier U, Meinel T, et al. Fluorescence-guided surgery with 5-aminolevulinic acid for resection of malignant glioma: a randomised controlled multicentre phase III trial. Lancet Oncol 2006;7(5):392–401.

26. Ruschel LG, Ramina R, da Silva EB Jr, et al. 5-Aminolevulinic acid fluorescence-guided surgery for spinal cord melanoma metastasis: a technical note. Acta Neurochir 2018;160(10):1905–8.

27. Zakaria S, Gamal-Eldeen AM, El-Daly SM, et al. Synergistic apoptotic effect of Doxil ® and aminolevulinic acid-based photodynamic therapy on human breast adenocarcinoma cells. Photodiagnosis Photodyn Ther 2014;11(2):227–38.

28. Tetard MC, Vermandel M, Mordon S, et al. Experimental use of photodynamic therapy in high grade gliomas: a review focused on 5-aminolevulinic acid. Photodiagnosis Photodyn Ther 2014;11(3):319–30.

29. Predina JD, Runge J, Newton A, et al. Evaluation of Aminolevulinic Acid-Derived Tumor Fluorescence Yields Disparate Results in Murine and Spontaneous Large Animal Models of Lung Cancer. Sci Rep 2019;9(1):7629.

30. Osaki T, Yokoe I, Ogura S, et al. Photodynamic detection of canine mammary gland tumours after oral administration of 5-aminolevulinic acid. Vet Comp Oncol 2017;15(3):731–9.

31. Osaki T, Gonda K, Murahata Y, et al. Photodynamic detection of a feline meningioma using 5-aminolaevulinic acid hydrochloride. JFMS Open Rep 2020;6(1). 2055116920907429.

32. Osaki T, Amaha T, Murahata Y, et al. Utility of 5-aminolaevulinic acid fluorescence-guided endoscopic biopsy for malignant mesothelioma in a cat and dog. Aust Vet J 2023;101(3):99–105.

Advances in Minimally Invasive Procedures of the Thoracic Cavity

Ingrid M. Balsa, MEd, DVM[a,b,*]

KEYWORDS

- Thoracoscopy • Minimally invasive surgery • Thymoma • One-lung ventilation
- Persistent right aortic arch • Lung lobectomy • Portoazygous shunt
- Thoracic drainage

KEY POINTS

- In dogs and cats the working space of the thoracic cavity may be increased by one-lung ventilation or insufflation of low-pressure carbon dioxide into the thoracic cavity.
- The thoracoscopic removal of small and medium-sized cranial mediastinal masses tends to be well tolerated in dogs. In dogs without myasthenia gravis, short and long-term outcomes are excellent with this approach.
- Thoracoscopic removal of medium-sized pulmonary masses and thoracoscopic lung lobectomies for a variety of other diseases have similar short and long-term outcomes to dogs undergoing thoracotomy.
- Patients with a persistent right aortic arch are routinely approached thoracoscopically for the transection of the ligamentum arteriosum. While the clinical significance of the role of the aberrant left subclavian artery remains disputed, the vessel can also be transected thoracoscopically.
- Thoracoscopic attenuation of portoazygous shunts is possible with ameroid ring constrictors and may allow for more optimal placement of the occlusion device than a celiotomy.

INTRODUCTION

With advances in minimally invasive surgery (MIS) and interventional radiology (IR) in veterinary medicine, there have been substantial gains in knowledge regarding minimally invasive procedures within the thoracic cavity, many of which have been covered in other chapters in this book. Discovery and the ability to advance these procedures seems to be occurring more quickly in our canine patients as compared with feline patients likely due to the size limitations of the feline thoracic cavity and the large

[a] Department of Clinical Sciences, Oregon State University, Corvallis, OR, USA; [b] Carlson College of Veterinary Medicine, 172 Magruder Hall, Corvallis, OR 97331, USA
* Corresponding author.
E-mail address: ingrid.balsa@oregonstate.edu

Vet Clin Small Anim 54 (2024) 697–706
https://doi.org/10.1016/j.cvsm.2024.02.005
vetsmall.theclinics.com

(human) size of much of the available minimally invasive equipment. As novel procedures are described, or historic procedures refined, it is essential to consider the anesthetic implications of working within the thoracic cavity. The various physiologic consequences of a pneumothorax while under general anesthesia are well outside the scope of this article. However, in addition to a pneumothorax, the avid thoracoscopic surgeon will soon be eager to attempt procedures that rely on the one-lung ventilation or carbon dioxide insufflation of the thoracic cavity to increase working space within the confines of the thorax. For this reason, as advances occur in minimally invasive procedures of the thoracic cavity it is equally as important to consider advances in the anesthetic management of these challenging clinical cases.

ONE-LUNG VENTILATION

The myriad of physiologic changes that occur during one-lung ventilation are far beyond the scope of this article or the expertise of the author. Perhaps more relevant to the small animal surgeon are the different devices used for and the various techniques described for assuring appropriate device placement for one-lung ventilation in dogs and cats.

As always with minimally invasive procedures, case selection, especially when in the early phases of the learning curve, are essential to success. Generally speaking, the left side of the lung field is easier to block than the right due to the relatively cranial location of the right cranial bronchus in dogs.

Devices

- Double-Lumen Endobronchial Tubes – most useful in dogs less than 30 kg due to length
  - Robert Shaw
  - Carlens
  - Dr. White
- Endobronchial Blockers – slower lung collapse compared with double-lumen tubes
  - Fogarty catheter – may be useful for dogs too large for Arndt endobronchial blocker
  - Arndt endobronchial blocker
  - EZ Blocker – forked, bilateral balloon ends, allows for alternating lung ventilation without repositioning the catheter

Techniques for Placement

Double-lumen tube or endobronchial blocker movement or dislodgement is a common occurrence in veterinary patients. Therefore, minimal movement of the patient's head and neck is recommended following the placement of the one-lung ventilation device. This means that it is optimal for placement to be done in the operating room with the patient positioned as it would be for surgery.

Blind placement of double-lumen tubes has been described by Mayhew and colleagues in 2012.[1] In this study, 3 different types of double-lumen tubes were evaluated with regards to achieving one-lung ventilation in healthy, purpose bred dogs. In this study the left-sided Robert Shaw tubes were the most likely to achieve one-lung ventilation both when initially placed and when repositioning manipulations were allowed under thoracoscopic guidance.[1]

Fluoroscopic-assisted placement of double-lumen tubes and bronchial blockers has been described in a canine cadaveric model.[2] This study found that both EZ blockers and Robert Shaw double-lumen tubes could be successfully placed using fluoroscopic guidance, with the left side being easier to block than the right. The EZ blockers were deemed slightly easier to place by the authors of the study, although the Robert Shaw tubes were slightly more successful in blocking the left lungs.[2]

Bronchoscopic-assisted placement of an endobronchial blocker is likely considered gold standard and may be necessary to fully block the right cranial bronchus in some dogs. In a cadaveric study by Mayhew and colleagues in 2019, bronchoscopic-assisted Arndt endobronchial blocker was successful in 100% of the dogs for both the right and left side.[2] In this study, the canine cadavers ranged in size from 20 to 37 kg. The endoscopists experience with bronchial anatomy and bronchial blockade likely influenced outcomes in this study.[2]

One-lung ventilation in cats seems to be even more challenging than in dogs, with blockade of the left side achieved in 5/6 cats and blockade of the right side only achieved in 2/6 cats even with bronchoscopic-assisted placement.[3] As in alternative, low-pressure thoracic carbon dioxide insufflation of 3 mm Hg has been investigated to improve the working space in the thorax of cats. This technique may be better tolerated in cats than in dogs due to the pliability of the feline thoracic wall.[3]

Carbon dioxide insufflation of the thoracic cavity, along with one-lung ventilation has also been described in healthy dogs. Pressure of 3 and 5 mm Hg were investigated, which showed an increased in working space volume when compared with one-lung ventilation alone.[4] Given the decrease in SpO_2 and ventilation space volume with an intrathoracic pressure of 5 mm Hg it is the author's opinion that no more than 3 mm Hg should be used in the thoracic cavity of dogs, and only if required and for as short a duration as possible.[4] Whenever carbon dioxide is insufflated into the thoracic cavity, intensive monitoring of patient blood pressure, heart rate, and patient oxygenation is required.

ETIOLOGY
Cranial Mediastinal Mass

The 2 most common types of cranial mediastinal masses in dogs and cats are lymphoma and thymic epithelial tumors. Preoperative diagnosis of the tumor is important since lymphoma is generally treated systemically, and thymic epithelial tumors are treated with local therapy, surgery, or radiation therapy. Diagnosis is most often achieved via ultrasound-guided fine needle aspirate. In dogs, appearance on thoracic radiographs or computed tomography (CT) may also assist with diagnosis, though ultimately at this time cytology is required. On canine thoracic radiographs, well defined mass margins and rightward displacement of the heart have been significantly associated with thymic epithelial tumors versus lymphoma.[5] No radiographic diagnostic criteria has been identified in cats. Historically, no diagnostic criteria had been identified on CT scan that differentiate the 2 neoplasias.[6] However more recently a standard deviation of greater than 17 Hounsfield units following IV contrast administration was significantly associated with thymic epithelial tumors when compared with lymphoma, likewise thymic epithelial tumors were less likely to envelop the cranial vena cava when compared with lymphoma.[7] When solely evaluating thymic epithelial tumors, CT findings such as increased tumor height and vascular invasion have been associated with recurrence.[8]

With considering thoracoscopy, a guideline for case selection proposed by a group of experienced minimally invasive surgeons is tumors less than 8 cm or 300 cm³ in dogs that are greater than 20 kg.[9] For this procedure, the patient is placed in dorsal recumbency, and one-lung ventilation is generally not required. In the most recent retrospective study, one-lung ventilation was only used in 16% of cases.[10] Subxiphoid cannula placement along with additional cannulas in both hemithorax with the monitor placed cranial to the patient's head will aid in triangulation. If pleural fluid is present, suctioning the fluid will allow for improved visualization by allowing the lungs to fall dorsally, away from the mass, which tend to be suspended in the mediastinum (**Fig. 1**). Dissection is generally performed with a combination of vessel sealing device and blunt dissection. In a more recent retrospective study by Carroll and colleagues, in 38 dogs that underwent thoracoscopic removal of cranial mediastinal masses, conversion to an open procedure was uncommon, happening in 11% of cases. The average tumor size in this case series was 4.9 cm with the maximum tumor diameter being 8.5 cm.[10]

Immediate and long-term postoperative outcomes may vary depending on if the dog has myasthenia gravis and concurrent megaesophagus at the time of surgery. In one study, these comorbidities were associated with decreased survival time compared with dogs without myasthenia gravis.[9] However, in a more recent study, myasthenia gravis did not affect median survival time.[10] Complications include emergent and nonemergency conversion to an open procedure, intraoperative hemorrhage, which may be life-threatening, and port site metastasis.[9,11] For this reason, removal of the mass using a specimen retrieval bag is of the utmost importance.

Lung Lobectomy

Video-assisted thoracoscopic surgery (VATS) and totally thoracoscopic lung lobectomy technique have been reported in dogs for the treatment of primary lung tumors, metastatic pulmonary lesions, pyothorax secondary to migrating foreign bodies, and lung lobe torsion.[12–16] Similar to cranial mediastinal masses, case selection for smaller masses (<7 cm), located toward the periphery of the lung lobe will be beneficial for thoracoscopic excision.[12–14] VATS lung lobectomy has been reported in dogs including tumor volumes up to 10 cm or 174.4 cm^3 being successfully resected.[14,17–20] VATS in cats is more common than thoracoscopic lung lobectomy due to the minimal working room within the thorax of a cat.

Thoracoscopic lung lobectomy takes place with the patient in lateral recumbency though the ability to rotate them into semi-sternal is helpful. Multiple port placements have been described with caudally placed ports more useful for cranial lung lobectomy

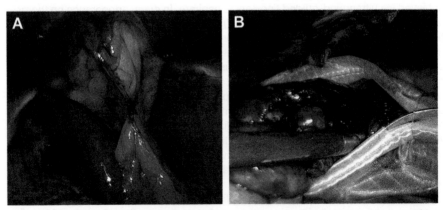

Fig. 1. Thoracoscopic view of a cranial mediastinal thymoma. (*A*) Thoracoscopic view of cranial mediastinal thymoma in a dog. (*B*) Thoracoscopic placement of thymoma into specimen retrival bag.

and cranially placed ports more useful for caudal lobectomy. One-lung ventilation is important in these procedures because it allows for better visualization of the mass and the hilus of the lung and increases the working space within the chest.[21] Optimal placement of the mini-thoracotomy in cats was described by Scott and colleagues in 2019 is summarized in **Table 1** later in discussion.[22]

Complications include conversion to open thoracotomy in 23% to 44% of cases.[12,13] Reasons for conversion include hemorrhage (intercostal artery), failure to achieve or maintain OLV, and poor access/visualization due to the location of the tumor.[12,13] Other complications include port site inflammation and infection; infection in these cases can extend into the thoracic cavity and result in pyothorax. There have been no significant differences in outcomes identified between dogs that had lung tumors removed via thoracoscopy or VATS or via open thoracotomy.[12,14]

Thoracoscopic lung biopsies have been described for diffuse pulmonary disease as well as small peripheral neoplastic masses. Loop ligatures, stapling devices, and vessel sealing devices have all been used for these procedures.[23,24] Additionally, ablation techniques for intrathoracic and suspected pulmonary metastatic lesions are an active area of research interest for many. Described techniques include video-assisted and percutaneous microwave ablation,[25,26] and radiofrequency ablation for chemodectomas.[27]

Persistent Right Aortic Arch

A variety of vascular ring anomalies have been reported in the veterinary literature with the most common clinically relevant vascular ring anomaly being a persistent right aortic arch. While there does appear to be some breed predisposition in German Shephard Dogs and Irish Setters, these anomalies can occur in any dog though they seem to be more common in large breed dogs and more common in dogs than in cats. In these patients the aortic arch is formed on the right side, from the vestigial right 4th arch, instead of the left 4th arch. Therefore, the ligamentum arteriosum encircles the esophagus before inserting in the main pulmonary artery. In addition to the ligamentum arteriosum creating a complete vascular ring in these patients, a number of these patients also have an aberrant left subclavian artery that arises from the right aortic arch and courses dorsally over the esophagus causing a second site of partial esophageal compression. Given the variety of vascular ring anomalies described in veterinary medicine, it is the author's belief that a CT angiogram is an essential preoperative diagnostic to accurately describe the cranial thoracic anatomy prior to considering a thoracoscopic approach to a patient with a suspected vascular ring anomaly.

| Table 1 | |
| Optimal placement of the mini-thoracotomy in cats | |
Lung Lobe	Optimal Intercostal Space for Mini-Thoracotomy
Left cranial	4–6
Left caudal	5&6
Right cranial/middle	4&5
Right caudal/accessory	5&6

Data from Scott, J. E., Singh, A., Case, J. B., Mayhew, P. D., & Runge, J. J. (2019). Determination of optimal location for thoracoscopic-assisted pulmonary surgery for lung lobectomy in cats. American Journal of Veterinary Research, 80(11), 1050-1054. Retrieved Jan 2, 2024, from https://doi.org/10.2460/ajvr.80.11.1050.

The first larger scale retrospective study to compare outcomes of dogs undergoing thoracotomy versus thoracoscopy for the transection of a left ligamentum arteriosum in dogs with persistent right aortic arches showed similar outcomes with regards to surgical times, complication types and rates, and postoperative time in the hospital.[28] However, this study had a relatively high conversion rate with one-third of the thoracoscopy patients being converted to thoracotomy. In this case series, patients were placed in right lateral recumbency, and the left hemithorax was explored via 3 to 4 cannulas placed in a variety of intercostal spaces from the 4th-11th space.[28]

A follow-up study on this topic looked at the need to perform one-lung ventilation in dogs undergoing the thoracoscopic transection of a ligamentum arteriosum. Of the 22 dogs in the study, 12 underwent one-lung ventilation with 10 dogs successfully having their ligamentum arteriosum transected whereas the remaining 10 dogs did not undergo one-lung ventilation and 7 dogs in this group had their ligamentum arteriosum transected. Interestingly in this study, 3 of the 5 converted dogs were converted due to hemorrhage, and only 2 of the dogs not undergoing one-lung ventilation were converted due to visualization.[29] It is unclear if one-lung ventilation in those cases would have allowed for the visualization of the ligamentum and safe transection without conversion. Unfortunately, due to the relatively small sample size in this study, it is difficult to draw conclusions as to the benefit of one-lung ventilation in these cases though it makes the case that one-lung ventilation is not required for the safe transection of a ligamentum arteriosum.

More recently, another small case series was published documenting the safe transection of the ligamentum arteriosum in dogs, as well as the transection of an aberrant left subclavian.[30] Because the aberrant left subclavian does not form complete vascular rings historically they have not routinely been transected although it is generally believed to be safe to do so. Nevertheless, there are anecdotal reports of dogs continuing to regurgitate following the transection of the ligamentum arteriosum which improve when the aberrant left subclavian is transected at a later date. For this reason, some surgeons consider the transection of the aberrant left subclavian, if present, as standard of care at the time of the initial surgery. Regardless, of when the transection occurs, it appears that the transection of an aberrant left subclavian less than 7 mm in diameter with a vessel-sealing device under thoracoscopic guidance is safe. In this case series of 5 dogs, one-lung ventilation was not used, and 2/5 dogs were converted to an open procedure, one due to poor visualization and one with a subclavian that exceeded 7 mm in diameter and therefore was suture ligated. Outcomes were good to excellent in these dogs with a median follow-up time of approximately 6 months.[30]

Porto-azygous Shunt Attenuation

Single, extrahepatic portosystemic shunts are common in small breed dogs and less common in large breed dogs and cats. Surgical attenuation of the shunts had been considered gold standard care with the ameroid ring constrictor being the preferred occlusion device due to allowing for gradual shunt occlusion. Laparoscopic treatment of single extrahepatic congenital shunts has been shown to be feasible in several studies.[31] In companion animals shunts are named depending on their vessel of origin and insertion. Shunts that insert on the azygous vein, portoazygous shunts, present a dilemma to the small animal surgeon in that the ideal placement of the ameroid ring constrictor, or other occlusion device, has always been around the shunt as close to shunt insertion on the systemic vasculature as possible to prevent missed branches of the shunt. The exception to this rule has been portoazygous shunts in which the occlusion device was placed on the shunt as cranial in the abdomen as possible.

Thoracic placement of a thin film cellophane band had been described by Casha and colleagues via a right lateral intercostal approach.[32] The outcome of the 3 dogs in the case series was good, with a decrease of serum bile acids by 8 weeks postoperative.[32] A transdiaphragmatic approach was described in both cadaveric and clinical patients by Or and colleagues[33] In this case series, thin film cellophane band were used in some patients and ameroid ring constrictors in others. Importantly, at follow-up, all dogs who had the placement of thin film cellophane bands required repeated surgery due to a lack of adhesions and fibrosis.[33] Therefore at this time, thin film cellophane banding cannot be recommended within the thoracic cavity. Nevertheless, some surgeons suggest that a thoracotomy is a more invasive procedure and is not justified in these cases. The ability to place an ameroid ring constrictor or cellophane band thoracoscopically has been evaluated in one cadaveric study.[34] In this study, access to the caudal azygous vein and placement of the occlusion devices were possible in all cadavers, ranging in size from 1.8 to 11 kg. A three cannula approach was used between rib spaces 9 to 11.[34] While exciting to consider in clinical patients, placement of the key in the ameroid ring constrictor in a live patient remains a challenging minimally invasive procedure.

Thoracic Effusions

Thoracic effusions in companion animals may occur for a variety of reasons causing patients to be presented for tachypnea, dyspnea, or respiratory distress. Thoracocentesis is often required to remove large volumes of thoracic fluid and allow for lung re-expansion. Complications of thoracocentesis include hemorrhage, pneumothorax, and pain. Generally speaking, patients need to be sedated in order to safely perform this procedure. For patients with chronic pleural effusions due to chylothorax unresponsive to surgical intervention or neoplastic effusions, placement of an intrathoracic drainage catheter (PlueralPort™) may allow for safer removal of the fluid, often without the need for sedation.

PleuralPorts have been used in both cats and dogs to manage chronic effusions and also allow for the instillation of intracavitary chemotherapeutic agents when appropriate.[35,36] These fenestrated silicone thoracostomy tubes allow for the long-term management of thoracic drainage or medication delivery via the subcutaneous port and Huber needle. Due to the subcutaneous port, the needle does not need to pass transthoracically, minimizing the risks typically associated with thoracocentesis. While historically PleuralPorts were placed at the time of surgical intervention (thoracotomy) for the primary disease or via a mini-thoracotomy approach both interventional radiologic and thoracoscopic descriptions of PleuralPort placement have been published.[36]

The placement of an intrathoracic drainage catheter using fluoroscopic guidance has been reported in both dogs and cats. A modified Seldinger technique was used with an over the needle catheter which allowed for the entry of a guidewire into the thoracic cavity. A peel-away sheath was then placed over the guidewire to allow for the introduction of the drainage catheter. This technique allowed for an alternative minimally invasive approach to intrathoracic drainage catheter placement.[37]

When being placed thoracoscopically general anesthesia is required, however if no other procedures are occurring at the same time it is unlikely that one-lung ventilation would be required to facilitate placement. The procedural description by Bianchi and colleagues involves the placement of two 6 mm cannula at the level of the 10th or 11th intercostal space. Thoracoscopic placement allows for the direct visualization of tube positioning and real-time adjustments can be made if needed. The benefit of thoracoscopic placement includes a visual evaluation of the hemithorax and biopsy of pleural lesions. The procedure time was 51 minutes.

While placement of intrathoracic drainage catheters is relatively straight forward, maintenance may not be, with the major complication being the obstruction of the catheter. Historically, catheters had been effective from 1 to 391 days.[35] In a more recent study, one port obstructed at Day 45; however, it was able to be flushed with sterile saline and return to function. In this case series, the median length of time that the ports were used was 5 months.[36]

While it appears that intrathoracic drainage catheter placement is well tolerated in dogs and cats as a medium-term solution, more information is needed regarding the optimal maintenance of these devices as well as the disease processes they may be best suited for.

SUMMARY

This article attempted to summarize some of the recent advances in minimally invasive thoracic procedures. There is no doubt that in the next decade there will be further refinement and advancement regarding these and other procedures. As discussed in other articles 3D printing and robotic surgery will likely alter the minimally invasive landscape. Collaborative research, advanced training opportunities such as the American College of Veterinary Surgeons MIS fellowship, and a desire to constantly improve care of patients will allow for continual growth in this exciting area of veterinary medicine.

CLINICS CARE POINTS

- One-lung ventilation of the right side (blocking of the left) is technically easier due to the anatomic configuration of the canine bronchial tree, specifically the cranial location of the right cranial bronchus,
- Canine mediastinal masses less than 8 cm and primary lung tumors less than 7 cm may be reasonable candidates for thoracoscopic removal
- Portoazygous shunt attenuation within the thoracic cavity should not be performed with thin film cellophane banding due to the lack of reliable adhesion formation.

DISCLOSURE

The author has nothing to disclose.

REFERENCES

1. Mayhew PD, Culp WT, Pascoe PJ, et al. Evaluation of blind thoracoscopic-assisted placement of three double-lumen endobronchial tube designs for one-lung ventilation in dogs. Vet Surg 2012;41(6):664–70.
2. Mayhew PD, Chohan A, Hardy BT, et al. Cadaveric evaluation of fluoroscopy-assisted placement of one-lung ventilation devices for video-assisted thoracoscopic surgery in dogs. Vet Surg 2020;49(Suppl 1):O93–101.
3. Mayhew PD, Pascoe PJ, Shilo-Benjamini Y, et al. Effect of One-Lung Ventilation With or Without Low-Pressure Carbon Dioxide Insufflation on Cardiorespiratory Variables in Cats Undergoing Thoracoscopy. Vet Surg 2015;44(Suppl 1):15–22.
4. Kanai E, Matsutani N, Watanabe R, et al. Effects of combined one-lung ventilation and intrathoracic carbon dioxide insufflation on intrathoracic working space when performing thoracoscopy in dogs. Am J Vet Res 2022;83(9):ajvr.

5. Oura TJ, Hamel PE, Jennings SH, et al. Radiographic differentiation of cranial mediastinal lymphomas from thymic epithelial tumors in dogs and cats. J Am Anim Hosp Assoc 2019 Jul/Aug;55(4):187–93.

6. Yoon J, Feeney DA, Cronk DE, et al. Computed tomographic evaluation of canine and feline mediastinal masses in 14 patients. Vet Radiol Ultrasound 2004;45(6): 542–6.

7. Reeve EJ, Mapletoft EK, Schiborra F, et al. Mediastinal lymphoma in dogs is homogeneous compared to thymic epithelial neoplasia and is more likely to envelop the cranial vena cava in CT images. Vet Radiol Ultrasound 2020;61:25–32.

8. von Stade L, Randall EK, Rao S, et al. CT imaging features of canine thymomas. Vet Radiol Ultrasound 2019;60(6):659–67.

9. MacIver MA, Case JB, Monnet EL, et al. Video-assisted extirpation of cranial mediastinal masses in dogs: 18 cases (2009–2014). J Am Vet Med Assoc 2017;250(11):1283–90.

10. Carroll KA, Mayhew PD, Culp WTN, et al. Thoracoscopic removal of cranial mediastinal masses in dogs: a retrospective case series of 38 dogs. Sorrento, Italy: Veterinary Endoscopy Society Meeting; 2023.

11. Alwen SGJ, Culp WTN, Szivek A, et al. Portal site metastasis after thoracoscopic resection of a cranial mediastinal mass in a dog. J Am Vet Med Assoc 2015; 247(7):793–800.

12. Bleakley S, Duncan CG, Monnet E. Thoracoscopic lung lobectomy for primary lung tumors in 13 dogs. Vet Surg 2015;44:1029–35.

13. Lansdowne JL, Monnet E, Twedt DC, et al. Thoracoscopic lung lobectomy for treatment of lung tumors in dogs. Vet Surg 2005;34:530–5.

14. Mayhew PD, Hunt GB, Steffey MA, et al. Evaluation of short-term outcome after lung lobectomy for resection of primary lung tumors via video-assisted thoracoscopic surgery or open thoracotomy in medium-to large-breed dogs. J Am Vet Med Assoc 2013;243:681–8.

15. Peláez MJ, Jolliffe C. Thoracoscopic foreign body removal and right middle lung lobectomy to treat pyothorax in a dog. J Small Anim Pract 2012;53:240–4.

16. Lee SY, Park SJ, Seok SH, et al. Thoracoscopic-assisted lung lobectomy using hem-o-lok clips in a dog with lung lobe torsion: a case report. Veterinární medicína 2014;59(6):315–8.

17. Dhumeaux MP, Haudiquet PR. Primary pulmonary osteosarcoma treated by thoracoscopy-assisted lung resection in a dog. Can Vet J 2009;50:755–8.

18. Laksito MA, Chambers BA, Yates GD. Thoracoscopic-assisted lung lobectomy in the dog: Report of two cases. Aust Vet J 2010;88:263–7.

19. Wormser C, Singhal S, Holt DE, et al. Thoracoscopic-assisted pulmonary surgery for partial and complete lung lobectomy in dogs and cats: 11 cases (2008–2013). J Am Vet Med Assoc 2014;245:1036–41.

20. Scott JE, Auzenne DA, Massari F, et al. Complications and outcomes of thoracoscopic-assisted lung lobectomy in dogs. Vet Surg 2023;52(1):106–15. https://doi.org/10.1111/vsu.13886.

21. Monnet E. Thoracoscopic Lung Biopsy and Lung Lobectomy. In: Fransson BA, Mayhew PD, editors. Small animal laparoscopy and thoracoscopy. Ames, IA, USA: ACVS Foundation and Wiley Blackwell; 2015. p. 287–93.

22. Scott JE, Singh A, Case JB, et al. Determination of optimal location for thoracoscopic-assisted pulmonary surgery for lung lobectomy in cats. Am J Vet Res 2019;80(11):1050–4.

23. Adamiak Z, Holak P, Piorek A. Thoracoscopic biopsy of lung tumors using a Roeder's loop in dogs. Pol J Vet Sci 2008;11:75–7.

24. Mayhew PD, Culp WT, Pascoe PJ, et al. Use of the Ligasure vessel-sealing device for thoracoscopic peripheral lung biopsy in healthy dogs. Vet Surg 2012;41: 523–8.
25. Dornbusch JA, Wavreille VA, Dent B, et al. Percutaneous microwave ablation of solitary presumptive pulmonary metastases in two dogs with appendicular osteosarcoma. Vet Surg 2020;49(6):1174–82.
26. Mazzaccari K, Boston SE, Toskich BB, et al. Video-assisted microwave ablation for the treatment of a metastatic lung lesion in a dog with appendicular osteosarcoma and hypertrophic osteopathy. Vet Surg 2017;46(8):1161–5.
27. Gómez Ochoa P, Alférez MD, de Blas I, et al. Ultrasound-Guided Radiofrequency Ablation of Chemodectomas in Five Dogs. Animals 2021;11(10):2790.
28. Nucci DJ, Hurst KC, Monnet E. Retrospective comparison of short-term outcomes following thoracoscopy versus thoracotomy for surgical correction of persistent right aortic arch in dogs. J Am Vet Med Assoc 2018;253(4):444–51.
29. Marvel SJ, Hafez A, Monnet E. Thoracoscopic treatment of persistent right aortic arch in dogs with and without one lung ventilation. Vet Surg 2022;51(S1): O107–17. https://doi.org/10.1111/vsu.13717.
30. Regier PJ, Case JB, Fox-Alvarez WA. Ligation of the ligamentum arteriosum and aberrant left subclavian artery in five dogs in which persistent right aortic arch had been diagnosed. Vet Surg 2021;50(Suppl 1):O26–31.
31. Poggi E, Rubio DG, Pérez Duarte FJ, et al. Laparoscopic portosystemic shunt attenuation in 20 dogs (2018-2021). Vet Surg 2022;51(S1):O138–49. https://doi.org/10.1111/vsu.13785.
32. Casha G, Jones C. Intercostal thoracotomy for surgical attenuation of portoazygos extrahepatic portosystemic shunts in three dogs: surgical technique and short-term outcomes. N Z Vet J 2022;70(6):332–9.
33. Or M, Kitshoff A, Devriendt N, et al. Transdiaphragmatic Approach to Attenuate Porto-Azygos Shunts Inserting in the Thorax. Vet Surg 2016;45(8):1013–8.
34. Carroll KA, Dickson RE, Scharf VF. Feasibility of thoracoscopic attenuation of the azygos vein as a model for portoazygos shunts: A canine cadaveric study. Vet Surg 2021;50:345–52.
35. Brooks AC, Hardie RJ. Use of the PleuralPort Device for Management of Pleural Effusion in Six Dogs and Four Cats. Vet Surg 2011;40:935–41.
36. Bianchi A, Collivignarelli F, Paolini A, et al. Thoracoscopic Assisted PleuralPort™ Application in Seven Dogs Affected by Chronic Pleural Effusion. Vet Sci 2023 Apr 29;10(5):324.
37. Gibson EA, Culp WTN. Fluoroscopic-guided placement of intra-thoracic drainage catheters and subcutaneous ports: procedural description and evaluation of short-term outcomes in dogs and cats. Veterinary Interventional Radiology and Interventional Endoscopy Society Meeting. May 2019;1-3.

Advances in the Treatment of Chylothorax

William Hawker, BVSc, MANZCVS*,
Ameet Singh, DVM, DVSc, DACVS (Small Animal)

KEYWORDS

- Idiopathic • Chylothorax • Lymphangiography • Near-infrared fluorescence
- Thoracoscopic • Canine • Feline

KEY POINTS

- Preoperative computed tomographic lymphangiography should be considered in all cases of idiopathic chylothorax to aid in surgical planning.
- Intraoperative lymphangiography with indocyanine green and near-infrared fluorescence allows for accurate intraoperative thoracic duct identification.
- Minimally invasive surgical techniques are associated with improved postoperative outcomes in dogs.

 Video content accompanies this article at http://www.vetsmall.theclinics.com.

INTRODUCTION
Definition

Chylothorax describes the accumulation of chyle, a milky fluid originating from the lymphatic system, within the thoracic cavity.[1,2] The accumulation of chyle invariably leads to respiratory difficulty, as well as chronic inflammatory changes to the lungs and heart.[3] Failure to achieve clinical resolution of chylothorax is frequently devastating, often resulting in euthanasia.

Anatomy/Pathophysiology

Chyle is produced in the small intestines during digestion. Chyle from the intestinal lymphatics, along with lymph from the liver and hindquarters is transported to an abdominal reservoir known as the cisterna chyli. Chyle is then transported to the thorax via the thoracic duct before emptying into the venous circulation at the level of the thoracic inlet.[3] Approximately a third of thoracic duct lymph flow originates in the liver in

Department of Clinical Studies, The Ontario Veterinary College, University of Guelph, 26 College Avenue West, Guelph, N1G 2W1, Ontario, Canada
* Corresponding author.
E-mail address: hawker@uoguelph.ca

Vet Clin Small Anim 54 (2024) 707–720
https://doi.org/10.1016/j.cvsm.2024.02.006
0195-5616/24/© 2024 Elsevier Inc. All rights reserved.

dogs and cats.[4,5] Additional lymphatics enter the thoracic duct from the left cranial half of the body. The thoracic duct variably anastomoses with the venous system via a valved structure at the left jugular, left subclavian, azygous vein, or vena cava. Drainage of the right cranial half of the body and peritoneum occurs separately via the right lymphatic duct and diaphragmatic lymphatics, respectively.

The cisterna chyli is a bipartite, saclike structure located in the retroperitoneal space dorsal to the aorta and is closely associated with the origins of the left renal and celiac arteries. In dogs with idiopathic chylothorax, the cisterna chyli often shows a comparatively complex anatomy with smaller and more numerous branching.[6,7] Thirteen percent of dogs with idiopathic chylothorax lack an identifiable cisterna.[8,9]

Similarly, the thoracic duct demonstrates variable anatomy, from multiple branches to a plexiform structure, although it typically lies dorsal to the aorta on the right in dogs and left in cats. At the level of entry into the thorax, the thoracic duct courses along the hypaxial musculature ventral to the sympathetic trunk and azygous vein. Branches are frequently identified contralateral to the "main" branch, complicating surgical occlusion and making accurate preoperative imaging essential.

Etiology

Logically, any disease that obstructs the normal flow of chyle may lead to "leakage" into the surrounding tissues, frequently the pleural space. Theoretically, increased central venous pressure has been postulated to contribute to disease through an elevation in hydrostatic pressure, although this has not been demonstrated.[10]

In companion animals, chylothorax is frequently considered idiopathic, although chylothorax in cats appears comparatively less common. Other reported etiologies include surgical trauma, neoplastic or fungal mass lesions of the cranial thorax, obstruction of the great veins in the cranial mediastinum, primary cardiac disease, pericardial effusion, trauma, and lung lobe torsions.[2,11–14] It is important to elucidate the primary etiology, as failure to address any underlying cause can frustrate surgical treatment. This article will focus primarily on the management of idiopathic chylothorax.

DISCUSSION
Diagnostic Approach

Primary workup in cases of suspected chylothorax should focus on confirmation of chylous effusion and a thorough evaluation for any predisposing conditions. Thoracocentesis facilitates effusion assessment, with elevated triglycerides compared to a paired serum sample consistent with chylous effusion. Effusion cholesterol levels are also typically less than that of serum. Cytologic evaluation can help to increase the index of suspicion for chylothorax but cell populations may vary.[15] Complete blood count, biochemical profile, heartworm testing, and urinalysis should be performed for minimum database. Additional testing may be required based on suspected patient comorbidities.

Abdominal and thoracic imaging is essential, with computed tomography (CT) ideal for the assessment of intrathoracic and abdominal structures. CT angiography should be performed to rule out intraluminal or extraluminal causes of venous obstruction. Echocardiography is recommended to screen for evidence of right-sided cardiac and constrictive pericardial disease. If constrictive pericardial disease is suspected based on echocardiography, cardiac catheterization and right atrial and ventricular pressure profilometry may be used for confirmation. Care must be taken to ensure accurate measurements are obtained, with potential variation due to equipment calibration, patient volume status, and anesthetic depth.

A recent study demonstrated a correlation between echocardiography results and the detection of constrictive pericardial physiology (CPP) based on cardiac catheterization in dogs. Using a mean right atrial pressure of 6 mm or greater as the gold standard for CPP diagnosis, echocardiography was shown to have a sensitivity of 94% and positive predictive value of 89%.[16] This may allow for less-invasive determination of CPP, aiding in preoperative planning (this is discussed in more detail in "Surgical technique selection"). However, care must be taken not to overinterpret results, with relatively low specificity (66%) of echocardiography in the detection of CPP in this same study.[16]

Computed tomographic lymphangiography
Computed tomographic lymphangiography (CTLA) is an essential component of chylothorax diagnosis and presurgical planning. CTLA allows for visualization of thoracic duct morphology, and delineation of duct branching that may alter surgical approach and/or technique (**Fig. 1**). Multiple methods of obtaining CTLA are described. Percutaneous injection of the mesenteric lymph nodes with 1.5 to 2 mL of nonionic iodinated contrast has shown good success in 2 case series.[15,17] Ultrasound guidance is required, and the lymph nodes must be ultrasonographically visible (at least 4–5 mm in diameter). Alternatively, a cut-down technique for the popliteal lymph node has been described. The patient is positioned in sternal on the CT table with the pelvic limbs pulled caudally to facilitate access. If sedated, local anesthesia can be infused in an inverted U pattern bilateral and proximal to the node. Approximately, a 4 cm skin incision typically allows nodal access, and administration of iohexol at a described dose of 60 mg of iodine per kilogram of body weight.[18,19] In instances of unsuccessful mesenteric or popliteal injection, alternate sites have been described, including perirectal, metatarsal region/pad, or percutaneous hepatic infusion.[20–23]

Obtaining good quality CTLA in cats can be more challenging. Chronic chylous effusion seems to be associated with a reduction in available lymph node size. A nodal width and length of at least 5 mm is likely required for successful popliteal or mesenteric lymph node injection. Successful CTLA was achieved in 7 out of 11 cats in one case series, with injection of the left and/or right hepatic lobes with 2 mL of iopamidol iodinated contrast (Isovue 370) under ultrasound guidance.[22]

Immediate postoperative CTLA (**Fig. 2**) has recently been advocated to ensure complete occlusion of the thoracic duct, as well as the absence of "sleeping" branches. Four of 19 (21%) dogs in which a diagnostic CTLA was performed immediately postoperatively showed evidence of residual flow in the thoracic duct in one study.[16] In 3 of

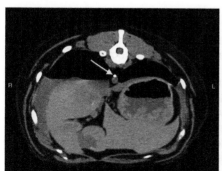 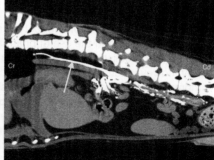

Fig. 1. Preoperative CTLA in a dog. The thoracic duct is delineated by the yellow arrow. Note the single duct at the level of the caudal thorax in this patient.

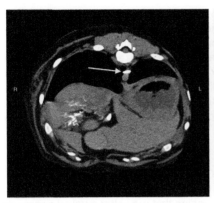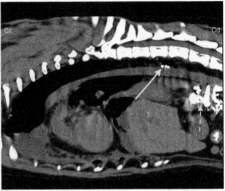

Fig. 2. Postoperative CTLA in a dog (same patient as **Fig. 1**). Endoscopic clips applied to the thoracic duct are indicated by the yellow arrow. These are in the caudal thorax at the location of the previously identified single thoracic duct on preoperative CTLA. Note the accumulation of contrast in the abdominal lymphatic system (*dashed blue arrow*) with the absence of forward flow through the thoracic duct, suggesting successful clip application.

these dogs, residual ducts were considered missed at the time of surgery, while the remaining dog showed multiple ducts not evident on preoperative CTLA consistent with "sleeping" branches.[16] Another study evaluated CTLA performed in dogs with idiopathic chylothorax 1 week postoperatively. This demonstrated the presence of "sleeping" branches in 4 out of 14 (28%) dogs, *without* the presence of chylothorax.[24] The clinical relevance of these "sleeping" branches remains undetermined, however, may represent a cause of treatment failure. Additionally, in instances of missed thoracic duct branches, immediate postoperative CTLA allows for direct surgical correction.

In cases of persistent chylous effusion, repeat CTLA allows for determination and classification of persistent thoracic duct flow. Interestingly, however, collateral duct formation or recanalization of the thoracic duct on routine postoperative CTLA does not necessarily equate to recurrence of chylous effusion. In one study, 5 out of 17 (29%) dogs showed evidence of persistent thoracic duct flow on 3 month postoperative CTLA, 2 of which were attributed to collateral duct formation, and 3 of which were attributed to recanalization of the thoracic duct.[16] Of these dogs, only 1 had suffered recurrence of chylous effusion at the time of publication.[16] The significance of these findings remains undetermined.

Medical Management

Medical management of chylothorax typically consists of intermittent drainage of the chest, low-fat diets, and the use of pharmaceuticals such as octreotide and rutin.[3]

There are no published guidelines as to what constitutes "failure" of conservative therapy; however, long-term, unresolved chylothorax can result in fibrosing pleuritis, pyothorax, and an increased septicemia risk.[2] As such, ongoing medical management is not typically recommended in the face of persistent disease.

Long-term drainage techniques have been described as alternatives to definitive surgical therapy. Pleuroperitoneal drains resulted in disease-free intervals of 20 months in one study, although drain-related complications were frequently reported.[25] Subcutaneous vascular access ports connected to pleural drains may be useful in instances of chronic serosanginous effusion following resolution of chylothorax. Their use in the long-term management of chylous effusion has been described but is often associated with early obstruction.[26] Long-term drainage may also result in dehydration, malnutrition, coagulation abnormalities, and electrolyte disturbances such as hyponatremia and hyperkalemia.[27,28] Careful monitoring is required if long-term drainage is pursued.

Surgical Management

Patient selection
Idiopathic chylothorax is generally considered a surgical disease. However, it is important to exclude other potential causes prior to surgical intervention. If traumatic chylothorax is suspected, intermittent thoracic drainage can be performed for 2 to 4 weeks to assess for spontaneous resolution. Similarly, care must be taken to rule out any predisposing factors. Failure to address the underlying cause in cases of secondary chylothorax has been associated with poor surgical outcomes, with only 2 of 5 dogs with nonidiopathic chylothorax demonstrating postsurgical resolution in one case series.[2]

Surgical technique selection
Surgical occlusion of the thoracic duct, or thoracic duct ligation (TDL), is the most commonly performed surgical procedure in the treatment of canine idiopathic chylothorax.[3] Occlusion of the thoracic duct encourages the formation of alternate chyle drainage tracts within the abdomen.[29,30] Theoretically, this should resolve thoracic fluid accumulation, although historical results of TDL alone have been poor with resolution rates of between 31% and 51%.[11,29–31] Additional interventions have been advocated in an attempt to improve surgical outcomes. These include subtotal pericardiectomy (SP) and cisterna chyli ablation (CCA).[11] Although, more recently, the necessity of these additional procedures has been challenged.[15,16]

Thoracic omentalization and pleuroperitoneal or pleurovenous shunts have also been described.[3,11,25,32] However, these have shown less-convincing clinical results, are not routinely used, or are reserved for refractory cases where more conventional techniques have failed.[3]

SP describes the removal of the pericardium to the level of the phrenic nerves bilaterally. Elevated venous pressures secondary to cardiac disease have been linked to chylothorax formation in dogs.[3] Chronic chylothorax irritates the pericardium, leading to pathologic changes, such as thickening.[1,10,30,32] It has been proposed that this thickening may contribute to persistently elevated venous pressures following TDL, predisposing to recurrent chylous effusion postoperatively.[1]

A 100% resolution rate in 10 dogs with idiopathic chylothorax in which both TDL and SP were performed concurrently (TDL-SP) was reported in one case series.[1] Subsequent literature confirmed the improvement in postoperative outcomes with TDL-SP, although resolution rates were varied.[2,12,15,30,31] A prospective randomized trial performed by McAnulty and colleagues, in 2011, showed only 60% resolution with TDL-SP, while a systematic review reported an overall clinical resolution rate of 74% when combining the results of 5 studies.[10,11]

More favorable results have been reported when using minimally invasive surgical techniques for the treatment of idiopathic chylothorax. In a multi-institutional retrospective study examining the outcome of 39 dogs undergoing thoracoscopic surgery for TDL-SP, 95% of patients showed resolution of chylous effusion, with only 3 dogs (9%) having recurrence.[15]

Recently, the role of pericardiectomy in the treatment of idiopathic chylothorax in the absence of CPP has been challenged. A prospective cohort study examining 26 dogs with idiopathic chylothorax used cardiac catheterization to determine the presence of CPP, defined as a mean right atrial pressure greater than 6 mm Hg and/or right ventricular end-diastolic pressure greater than 10 mm Hg.[16] Using thoracoscopy, TDL-SP was only performed in instances of confirmed CPP, otherwise TDL was performed alone. No difference in outcome was observed between groups with resolution rates of 94% and 88% for TDL and TDL-SP, respectively (**Table 1**).[16] It was concluded that SP may only be required in instances of confirmed CPP. Resolution rates with TDL alone were also much higher than previously reported; however, postoperative CTLA were performed in 92% of cases with persistent thoracic duct flow observed in 4 dogs, 3 of which were returned immediately to surgery for repeated occlusion.[16] Detection and immediate treatment of missed ducts at the time of surgery may have contributed to the improved outcomes observed in this cohort. Nevertheless, based on these results, it may be feasible to consider thoracoscopic TDL alone in cases where there is no evidence of CPP.

Surgical destruction of the abdominal chyle reservoir, or CCA, has been suggested as an alternate adjunct to TDL in the treatment of idiopathic chylothorax. Sicard and colleagues, in 2005, suggested that failure of TDL was likely due to the formation of new lymphatic channels into the chest, bypassing the original site of surgical occlusion.[29] This, they proposed, was secondary to high pressures within the thoracic duct following ligation, encouraging the recruitment of these alternate pathways.[29] As the primary source of chyle draining into the thoracic duct, it was hoped that by surgically destroying the cisterna chyli, this pressure would be relieved—thereby reducing the likelihood of disease recurrence.[29] In the initial pilot study by the same authors, 5 out of the 6 dogs treated by combined TDL and CCA (TDL-CCA) demonstrated appropriate formation of new chyle drainage tracts within the abdomen.[29] However, this study was conducted under experimental conditions, making extrapolation to clinical cases challenging. Data on TDL-CCA outcomes remain limited, although in a randomized prospective trial, TDL-CCA was associated with improved resolution rates (83%) as compared to traditional TDL-SP (60%).[10] Due to the small sample size, statistical significance was not reached.

Table 1
Summary of results for patients undergoing thoracoscopic thoracic duct ligation with or without pericardiectomy dependent on the diagnosis of constrictive pericardial pathology

	TDL	TDL/P[a]	P-value
Echocardiography score ≥2[b]	1/17 (6%)	6/9 (67%)	—
Mean right atrial pressure (mm Hg)	4.2 (1.7–5.9)	6.4 (6.1–11.6)	—
Mean right ventricular end-diastolic pressure (mm Hg)	6.8 (1.8–9)	10 (6.3–14.5)	—
Incomplete TDL at 3 mo postoperative CTLA	4/13 (31%)	1/4 (25%)	.56
Perioperative mortality	0/17 (0%)	1/9 (11%)	.35
Resolution rate	16/17 (94%)	7/8 (88%)	.55
Late recurrence rate	1/17 (6%)	0/8 (0%)	.71

[a] Either SP or pericardial window with fillets performed in conjunction with TDL.
[b] Score based on the evaluation of echocardiographic cine loops. One point was given for the presence of each of the following: right atrial enlargement, septal bounce, pericardial thickening, and caval and hepatic vein enlargement.

Data from: Mayhew, P. D., Balsa, I. M., Stern, J. A., Johnson, E. G., Kaplan, J., Gonzales, C., Steffey, M. A., Gibson, E., Hagen, B., Culp, W. T. N., & Giuffrida, M. (2023). Resolution, recurrence, and chyle redistribution after thoracic duct ligation with or without pericardiectomy in dogs with naturally occurring idiopathic chylothorax. Journal of the American Veterinary Medical Association, 261(5), 696–704. https://doi.org/10.2460/javma.22.08.0381

While both the combination of TDL-SP and TDL-CCA show promise, the clinical data remain limited. The majority of the veterinary literature is retrospective in nature and is limited to small case series.[11] A systematic review by Reeves and colleagues in 2019 concluded, "there was limited quality and quantity of data to support one treatment over another for IC [idiopathic chylothorax] in dogs and cats." In this same review, only one study examining idiopathic chylothorax in dogs was found to have a higher level of evidence based on assessment by the GRADE and Oxford Level of Evidence classification schemes.[11]

Mayhew and colleagues, in 2023, have more recently challenged the necessity of combining TDL with SP and/or CCA.[16] It is clear, in select cases, that resolution of chylothorax can be achieved with TDL alone. This is likely reflective of improved perioperative imaging and advancements in surgical technique. The advent of minimally invasive surgical techniques and near-infrared fluorescence (NIRF) imaging has revolutionized the surgical treatment of chylothorax. These are outlined in more detail in the "Surgical advances" section.

Data surrounding the treatment of feline chylothorax are even more limited, but it is generally accepted that cats have a poorer outcome than dogs regardless of surgical technique, although long-term resolution can be accomplished.[33,34]

Surgical advances

Intraoperative duct visualization. Intraoperative methylene blue lymphangiography has traditionally been used for thoracic duct visualization during surgery. Methylene blue is diluted with 1:10 saline and administered at a dose of 1 mL per dog and 0.1 mL per cat. Direct injection into the ileocecocolic lymph node is preferred over popliteal lymph node injection, and requires a limited paracostal abdominal approach.[15] Duration of coloration may vary between patients, but it is expected to last between 10 and 60 minutes.[35] It is the authors' experience, however, that coloration lasts for a much shorter period of time and reinjection is commonly required.

More recently, the use of NIRF imaging following the injection of indocyanine green (ICG) has emerged as a useful tool to aid in the identification of the thoracic duct (**Fig. 3**). Improved visibility of lymphatic branching has been reported with the use of NIRF as compared to methylene blue.[7] Use of NIRF also affords flexibility in

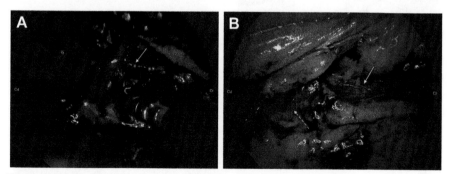

Fig. 3. Intraoperative visualization of the thoracic duct using NIRF with perirectal ICG administration. (*A*) Pre-TDL. The yellow arrow denotes the thoracic duct. The ease of identification facilitated by NIRF is evident. More caudally, there is branching of the TDL (dashed blue *arrow*), and this may be a less desirable location for endoscopic clip application. (*B*) Post-TDL with endoscopic clips (yellow *arrow*). Continued fluorescence of the thoracic duct is evident caudally, but no forward flow of fluorescence is visualized, indicative of successful clip application.

injection location, with successful fluorescence of the duct reported using efferent mesenteric lymphatics, perirectal and intrahepatic injection.[7,36,37] Alternate injection portals may eliminate the requirement for a paracostal abdominal approach, minimizing surgical time. The authors have had excellent success utilizing the perirectal technique for ICG injection. Submucosal ICG injection is performed immediately cranial to the anocutaneous line in a 4 quadrant pattern (**Fig. 4**). This can be performed during surgical preparation, approximately 20 to 30 minutes prior to the start of surgery. Doses of 0.25 - 1 ml of a 0.25 mg/ml diluted solution of ICG per quadrant have achieved reliable thoracic duct visualization.

Minimally invasive intervention. Thoracoscopic surgery has been used successfully to perform TDL, SP, and CCA. Outcomes with thoracoscopic TDL-SP have been favorable, particularly with the improvement in preoperative imaging (CTLA) and intraoperative duct identification (NIRF). Resolution rates in 2 recent studies with the use of thoracoscopic TDL-SP were 94% and 88%, respectively.[15,16] Interestingly, in the latter study, when TDL was performed without SP in the absence of CPP, a resolution rate of 94% was achieved in 17 dogs (see **Table 1**).[16] These studies highlight the success of minimally invasive intervention, with favorable results compared to those historically reported with open surgery.[11] They also question the benefit of SP in patients with no evidence of cardiac pathology. In dogs with no evidence of CPP on preoperative echocardiography, it may be feasible to perform thoracoscopic TDL without SP, avoiding additional surgical risks and patient morbidity while also reducing surgical time.

Thoracoscopic TDL is typically performed with the animal in sternal or lateral oblique recumbency (**Fig. 5**). Most frequently, a right-sided approach is performed in dogs and left-sided in cats; however, preoperative CTLA should be used to determine the optimal side. The targeted intercostal space in the caudal thorax for the placement

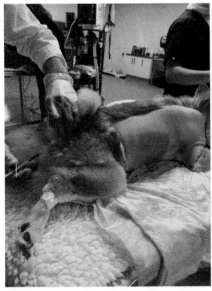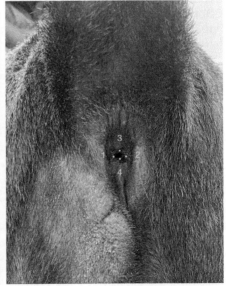

Fig. 4. Perirectal injection of ICG as performed at the authors' institution. Submucosal injection is performed in 4 quadrants (*blue dots*) just cranial to the anocutaneous line (*red dashed line*).

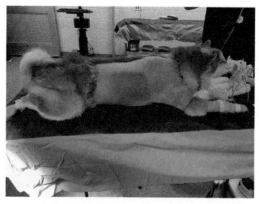

Fig. 5. A patient positioned in sternal recumbency in preparation for TDL. Padded support should be placed under the sternum and pubis to prevent obstruction of lymphatic flow, which may impede intraoperative identification of the thoracic duct.

of camera and instrument portals is ideally at a location of minimal duct branching based on preoperative CTLA. Frequently, portals are placed at the 9th, 10th, and 11th intercostal spaces (**Fig. 6**). Dissection of the thoracic duct and endoscopic clip application are shown in Videos 1 and 2, respectively.

If preoperative CTLA is unavailable, en bloc duct ligation may be required to ensure adequate ligation of all duct branches. En bloc ligation should encompass the entire mediastinum dorsal, ventral, and lateral to the aorta and can be performed thoracoscopically. An alternate technique for en bloc ligation was recently described in which ligation using intracorporeal sutures of all structures dorsal to the aorta, including the azygous vein, was initially performed, followed by separate ligation of the ventral mediastinum.[38] Long-term resolution of chylothorax was reported in 6 out of 7 (85.7%) dogs using this method.[38]

Thoracoscopic pericardiectomy is performed using a subxiphoid camera portal, with additional instrument portals placed in the caudal ventral intercostal spaces

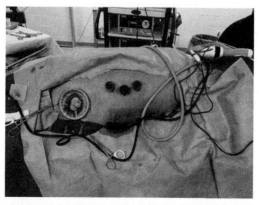

Fig. 6. Typical port placement for thoracoscopic TDL. A limited paracostal approach for intraoperative methylene blue lymphangiography has also been performed in this instance. Placement of a wound retraction device allows for easy exteriorization of the ileocecocolic lymph node.

as required. Care should be taken if using electrosurgical devices, as cardiac arrhythmias have been reported.[15,39] Different pericardiectomy techniques have been described including SP, modified SP, and pericardial window with vertical fillets.[15,39,40] Pericardial fillet and modified SP are beneficial in instances where visualization, particularly of the dorsal aspect of the pericardium, is challenging and 1-lung ventilation is not possible or desired.[35,39,40] A direct comparison of these techniques has not been performed, although all have reported successful outcomes when combined with TDL.[15]

Laparoscopic CCA is performed with the patient in sternal recumbency. Single and multiport techniques have been described.[41,42] The side of abdominal approach is ideally determined based on the location of the cisterna chyli on preoperative CTLA, although a left-sided approach may be preferable to avoid the vena cava during dissection. Laparoscopic CCA is shown in Video 3. While feasibility studies have been performed, no studies have evaluated long-term clinical outcomes in animals treated with laparoscopic CCA for idiopathic chylothorax.[41,42]

Thoracic duct embolization has been suggested as an alternative to CCA. Efferent mesenteric lymphatic vessel catheterization for embolic solution administration has been described via open abdominal surgery and a limited paracostal approach.[43–45] Percutaneous catheterization and embolization of the thoracic duct was found to be feasible in one study but was technically challenging and not recommended for clinical use.[46] In a prospective case series, a good clinical outcome, as defined by clinical resolution of chylous effusion, was achieved in 5 out of 6 dogs in which thoracoscopic TDL-SP and lymphatic embolization was performed.[43] Embolization was performed using a mixture of 3:1 lipiodol:n-butyl cyanoacrylate embolic solution under fluoroscopic guidance.[43] Successful catheterization of an efferent mesenteric lymphatic was unable to be performed in 2 smaller patients in this study.[43] Additional cohorts are required to determine the future role and feasibility of thoracic duct embolization in the treatment of canine chylothorax.

SUMMARY
Future Directions

The development of minimally invasive techniques has allowed for a reduction in perioperative morbidity in the treatment of chylothorax in companion animals. Determination as to the ideal procedure/s for the treatment of chylothorax, however, remains elusive. Recent literature describing the use of thoracoscopic TDL + SP has shown promising results compared to traditional open surgery. More recently, the role of SP in dogs not suffering from CPP has come into question. Thoracoscopic TDL as a sole treatment may be the ideal course of action in dogs without CPP and would leave a minimal surgical footprint. Laparoscopic CCA has been shown to be technically feasible; however, long-term clinical studies evaluating its role in the treatment of idiopathic chylothorax are lacking. Additional research is required to determine the exact role that SP, CCA, and thoracic duct embolization should play in the treatment of chylothorax. Large, prospective, randomized trials should be considered to further investigate surgical treatment. Unfortunately, due to the relative infrequency of disease, this may be technically challenging and/or require multi-institutional collaboration.

The increasing use of NIRF represents an exciting development in the treatment of chylothorax. Optimal dosing concentration and location should be investigated to aid in surgical duct visualization. Techniques to determine complete TDL more accurately at the time of surgery may aid in the prevention of treatment failure and warrant additional investigation.

Finally, despite the advances in idiopathic chylothorax treatment, the underlying disease process remains poorly defined. As diagnostic abilities improve, additional investigation as to the pathophysiology of this disease will aid future treatment directions.

Conclusions

Surgical treatment for canine idiopathic chylothorax has significantly evolved since the earliest reports of intervention. The advent of advanced imaging (CTLA) and NIRF have facilitated a shift toward less-invasive surgical techniques, with an associated improvement in clinical outcomes. While the ideal combination of procedures remains undetermined, excellent clinical outcomes can be achieved with thoracoscopic TDL alone in the absence of constrictive pericardial pathology. Feline chylothorax remains a more challenging clinical conundrum where success rates are still not as favourable as in canine patients.

CLINICS CARE POINTS

- Preoperative CT lymphangiography (CTLA) is considered an essential component of preoperative planning as it allows for accurate assessment of duct morphology but can be challenging in cats.

- Intraoperative lymphangiography aids accurate duct identification and dissection. NIRF appears superior to methylene blue for duct identification.

- Pericardiectomy (SP), CCA, and thoracic duct embolization are described as adjunctive procedures to TDL. The ideal combination of procedures remains undetermined, although TDL-SP shows the most evidence.

- Thoracoscopic surgery has shown excellent clinical outcomes when used to perform TDL-SP.

- In the absence of constrictive pericardial pathology, excellent clinical outcomes may be achieved with thoracoscopic TDL alone.

DISCLOSURE

There are no other financial or institutional disclosures related to this research.

SUPPLEMENTARY DATA

Supplementary data related to this article can be found online at https://doi.org/10.1016/j.cvsm.2024.02.006.

REFERENCES

1. Fossum TW, Mertens MM, Miller MW, et al. Thoracic duct ligation and pericardectomy for treatment of idiopathic chylothorax. J Vet Intern Med 2004;18(3):307–10.
2. Allman DA, Radlinsky MG, Ralph AG, et al. Thoracoscopic thoracic duct ligation and thoracoscopic pericardectomy for treatment of chylothorax in dogs. Vet Surg 2010;39(1):21–7.
3. Singh A, Brisson B, Nykamp S. Idiopathic chylothorax in dogs and cats: Nonsurgical and surgical management. Compendium 2012;34(8):E3.
4. Mobley WP, Kintner K, Witte CL, et al. Contribution of the liver to thoracic duct lymph flow in a motionless subject. Lymphology 1989;22(2):81–4.
5. Morris B. The hepatic and intestinal contributions to the thoracic duct lymph. Q J Exp Physiol Cogn Med Sci 1956;41(3):318–25.

6. Rengert R, Wilkinson T, Singh A, et al. Morphology of the cisterna chyli in nine dogs with idiopathic chylothorax and in six healthy dogs assessed by computed tomographic lymphangiography. Vet Surg 2021;50(1):223–9.

7. Steffey MA, Mayhew PD. Use of direct near-infrared fluorescent lymphography for thoracoscopic thoracic duct identification in 15 dogs with chylothorax. Vet Surg 2018;47(2):267–76.

8. Birch S, Barberet V, Bradley K, et al. Computed tomographic characteristics of the cisterna chyli in dogs. Vet Radiol Ultrasound 2014;55(1):29–34.

9. Johnson VS, Seiler G. Magnetic resonance imaging appearance of the Cisterna chyli. Vet Radiol Ultrasound 2006;47(5):461–4.

10. McAnulty JF. Prospective Comparison of Cisterna Chyli Ablation to Pericardectomy for Treatment of Spontaneously Occurring Idiopathic Chylothorax in the Dog. Vet Surg 2011;40(8):926–34.

11. Reeves LA, Anderson KM, Luther JK, et al. Treatment of idiopathic chylothorax in dogs and cats: A systematic review. Vet Surg 2020;49(1):70–9.

12. Carobbi B, White RaS, Romanelli G. Treatment of idiopathic chylothorax in 14 dogs by ligation of the thoracic duct and partial pericardiectomy. Vet Rec 2008;163(25):743–5.

13. Birchard SJ, McLoughlin MA, Smeak DD. Chylothorax in the dog and cat: A review. Lymphology 1995;28(2):64–72.

14. Fossum TW, Birchard SJ, Jacobs RM. Chylothorax in 34 dogs. J Am Vet Med Assoc 1986;188(11):1315–8.

15. Mayhew PD, Steffey MA, Fransson BA, et al. Long-term outcome of video-assisted thoracoscopic thoracic duct ligation and pericardectomy in dogs with chylothorax: A multi-institutional study of 39 cases. Vet Surg 2019;48(S1): O112–20.

16. Mayhew PD, Balsa IM, Stern JA, et al. Resolution, recurrence, and chyle redistribution after thoracic duct ligation with or without pericardiectomy in dogs with naturally occurring idiopathic chylothorax. J Am Vet Med Assoc 2023;261(5): 696–704.

17. Johnson EG, Wisner ER, Kyles A, et al. Computed tomographic lymphography of the thoracic duct by mesenteric lymph node injection. Vet Surg 2009;38(3): 361–7.

18. Lee N, Won S, Choi M, et al. CT thoracic duct lymphography in cats by popliteal lymph node iohexol injection. Vet Radiol Ultrasound 2012;53(2):174–80.

19. Singh A, Brisson BA, Nykamp S, et al. Comparison of computed tomographic and radiographic popliteal lymphangiography in normal dogs. Vet Surg 2011; 40(6):762–7.

20. Lin L-S, Chiu H-C, Nishimura R, et al. Computed tomographic lymphangiography via intra-metatarsal pad injection is feasible in dogs with chylothorax. Vet Radiol Ultrasound 2020;61(4):435–43.

21. Kim K, Cheon S, Kang K, et al. Computed tomographic lymphangiography of the thoracic duct by subcutaneous iohexol injection into the metatarsal region. Vet Surg 2020;49(1):180–6.

22. Johnson EG, Mayhew PD, Runge JJ. Computed tomographic lymphangiography following percutaneous intrahepatic injection of iopamidol in cats. Am J Vet Res 2023;84(2). ajvr.22.08.0147.

23. Ando K, Kamijyou K, Hatinoda K, et al. Computed tomography and radiographic lymphography of the thoracic duct by subcutaneous or submucosal injection. J Vet Med Sci 2012;74(1):135–40.

24. Kanai H, Furuya M, Yoneji K, et al. Canine idiopathic chylothorax: Anatomic characterization of the pre- and postoperative thoracic duct using computed tomography lymphography. Vet Radiol Ultrasound 2021;62(4):429–36.

25. Smeak DD, Stephenj null, Birchard null, et al. Treatment of chronic pleural effusion with pleuroperitoneal shunts in dogs: 14 cases (1985-1999). J Am Vet Med Assoc 2001;219(11):1590–7.

26. Brooks AC, Hardie RJ. Use of the PleuralPort device for management of pleural effusion in six dogs and four cats. Vet Surg 2011;40(8):935–41.

27. Attar MA, Donn SM. Congenital chylothorax. Semin Fetal Neonatal Med 2017; 22(4):234–9.

28. Willard MD, Fossum TW, Torrance A, et al. Hyponatremia and hyperkalemia associated with idiopathic or experimentally induced chylothorax in four dogs. J Am Vet Med Assoc 1991;199(3):353–8.

29. Sicard GK, Waller KR, McAnulty JF. The Effect of Cisterna Chyli Ablation Combined with Thoracic Duct Ligation on Abdominal Lymphatic Drainage. Vet Surg 2005;34(1):64–70.

30. da Silva CA, Monnet E. Long-term outcome of dogs treated surgically for idiopathic chylothorax: 11 cases (1995-2009). J Am Vet Med Assoc 2011;239(1): 107–13.

31. Stewart K, Padgett S. Chylothorax treated via thoracic duct ligation and omentalization. J Am Anim Hosp Assoc 2010;46(5):312–7.

32. Bussadori R, Provera A, Martano M, et al. Pleural omentalisation with en bloc ligation of the thoracic duct and pericardiectomy for idiopathic chylothorax in nine dogs and four cats. Vet J 2011;188(2):234–6.

33. Haimel G, Liehmann L, Dupré G. Thoracoscopic en bloc thoracic duct sealing and partial pericardectomy for the treatment of chylothorax in two cats. J Feline Med Surg 2012;14(12):928–31.

34. Stockdale SL, Gazzola KM, Strouse JB, et al. Comparison of thoracic duct ligation plus subphrenic pericardiectomy with or without cisterna chyli ablation for treatment of idiopathic chylothorax in cats. J Am Vet Med Assoc 2018;252(8):976–81.

35. Fransson BA, Singh A, Mayhew PD. Minimally Invasive Treatment of Chylothorax. In: Fransson BA, Mayhew PD, editors. Small animal laparoscopy and thoracoscopy. Hoboken, NJ, USA: John Wiley & Sons, Ltd; 2022. p. 385–99.

36. Korpita MF, Mayhew PD, Steffey MA, et al. Thoracoscopic detection of thoracic ducts after ultrasound-guided intrahepatic injection of indocyanine green detected by near-infrared fluorescence and methylene blue in dogs. Vet Surg 2022;51(S1): O118–27.

37. Kamijo K, Kanai E, Oishi M, et al. Perirectal injection of imaging materials for computed tomographic lymphography and near infrared fluorescent thoracoscopy in cats. Veterinární Medicína 2019;64(8):342–7.

38. Kanai H, Furuya M, Hagiwara K, et al. Efficacy of en bloc thoracic duct ligation in combination with pericardiectomy by video-assisted thoracoscopic surgery for canine idiopathic chylothorax. Vet Surg 2020;49(S1):O102–11.

39. Barbur LA, Rawlings CA, Radlinsky MG. Epicardial exposure provided by a novel thoracoscopic pericardectomy technique compared to standard pericardial window. Vet Surg 2018;47(1):146–52.

40. Mayhew KN, Mayhew PD, Sorrell-Raschi L, et al. Thoracoscopic subphrenic pericardectomy using double-lumen endobronchial intubation for alternating one-lung ventilation. Vet Surg 2009;38(8):961–6.

41. Sakals S, Schmiedt CW, Radlinsky MG. Comparison and description of trans-diaphragmatic and abdominal minimally invasive cisterna chyli ablation in dogs. Vet Surg 2011;40(7):795–801.

42. Morris KP, Singh A, Holt DE, et al. Hybrid single-port laparoscopic cisterna chyli ablation for the adjunct treatment of chylothorax disease in dogs. Vet Surg 2019; 48(S1):O121–9.

43. Carvajal JL, Case JB, Vilaplana Grosso FR, et al. Prospective evaluation of lymphatic embolization as part of the treatment in dogs with presumptive idiopathic chylothorax. Vet Surg 2022;51(S1):O128–37.

44. Pardo AD, Bright RM, Walker MA, et al. Transcatheter Thoracic Duct Embolization in the Dog An Experimental Study. Vet Surg 1989;18(4):279–85.

45. Clendaniel DC, Weisse C, Culp WTN, et al. Salvage Cisterna Chyli and Thoracic Duct Glue Embolization in 2 Dogs with Recurrent Idiopathic Chylothorax. J Vet Intern Med 2014;28(2):672.

46. Singh A, Brisson BA, O'Sullivan ML, et al. Feasibility of percutaneous catheterization and embolization of the thoracic duct in dogs. AJVR 2011;72(11):1527–34.

Augmenting Veterinary Minimally Invasive Surgery

Evidence-based Review of Foundational and Novel Devices and Technology

Erin A. Gibson, DVM, DACVS-SA

KEYWORDS

- Articulating instrumentation • Novel imaging platforms • Single-incision
- Valveless cannula • Endoscopic stapler • Hemostatic technology

KEY POINTS

- A substantial focus on enhancing and improving the accurate, unobstructed view of the surgical field in minimally invasive surgery has led to developments in 3 dimensional and 4K ultrahigh-definition technology, antifog and smoke evacuation systems, and wide-view laparoscopy.
- A novel application of single-incision devices continues to expand in veterinary medicine, including utility in retroperitoneoscopy and transanal access platforms.
- There is an increased understanding of the utility and reusability of hemostatic devices capable of navigating a minimally invasive surgical field such as bipolar and ultrasonic vessel-sealing devices, pretied ligature loops, and endoscopic staplers.
- Nonmechanized articulating instrumentation may provide improved dexterity and degrees of freedom to minimally invasive surgery that was previously exclusively available to robotic surgery.
- The evidence-based performance of new and older technologies is key to understanding clinical utility and impact on patient outcomes.

INTRODUCTION

The first laparoscopic and thoracoscopic platforms were developed in the 1980s and 1990s, and since then, technologic advances in the field of minimally invasive surgery (MIS) remain essential to the progress, success, and breadth of procedures performed. Veterinary MIS is unique in that purpose-made instrumentation and technology is rare, and more often than not, veterinary surgeons are applying medical devices suited for adult or pediatric human patients, which can incompletely address the needs of the

University of Pennsylvania, Matthew J. Ryan Veterinary Hospital, Department of Clinical Sciences and Advanced Medicine, 3900 Delancey Street, Philadelphia, PA 19104, USA
E-mail address: eagibson@upenn.edu

Vet Clin Small Anim 54 (2024) 721–733
https://doi.org/10.1016/j.cvsm.2024.02.007
0195-5616/24/© 2024 Elsevier Inc. All rights reserved.

veterinarian. The purpose of this review is to identify novel instrumentation and technology as well as to provide an updated purview of the novel role and utility of new, and old, devices, in veterinary MIS. Specifically, articulating instruments, cannulas, and electrosurgical, stapling, and ligating devices are discussed. Finally, imaging technology including 3D and 4K technology and wide-view laparoscopy will be discussed.

ARTICULATING INSTRUMENTS

While robotic surgery advances in the field of human medicine, the advantages of mechanized instruments with multiple degrees of freedom (DOF) have translated into the novel use of robotic devices also in standard laparoscopy. These include the multi-DOF articulating devices such as ArtiSential instruments (LivsMed, Seongnam, Korea) and FlexDex (FD) needle grasper (FlexDex Surgical, Brighton, MI).[1] The theoretic advantages, once the learning curve for these nonmechanized devices has been overcome, are in improved dexterity comparable to robotic and mechanized instruments without the associated cost (Fig. 1). In single-incision and multiport laparoscopic gastrectomy, the ArtiSential graspers and dissectors were considered a feasible alternative to standard instrumentation[2,3] and performed comparably to the da Vinci robot in a challenging suturing task[4] and in clinical gastrectomy.[5]

To the knowledge of the author, evidence of clinical experience using the FD device has not yet been published. In simulated suture models, the FD device allowed completion of difficult suturing tasks by novice surgeons more effectively and ergonomically compared to standard instrumentation.[6] Conversely, significantly longer task completion times and greater errors were identified in another study with the FD.[7] The author has had positive clinical experiences with this device in intracorporeal suturing for laparoscopic gastropexy in dogs, although evidence of superiority of this device over standard rigid instrumentation is lacking. Further clinical use of these instruments will be essential to better understand potential benefits and appropriate case selection for optimization of their advantages (multi-DOF) over rigid instrumentation.

SINGLE-INCISION LAPAROSCOPY DEVICES

Single-incision access systems have been utilized in veterinary medicine over the past decade for a variety of procedures. The single-incision access platforms enable

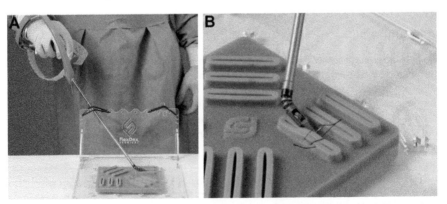

Fig. 1. (A) Articulating nonmechanized needle driver (FlexDex) device demonstrated on nonsurgical platform. (B) Needle driver performing in simulation of simple continuous suture line using articulating head for appropriate driving angle. (Used with permission from FlexDex Surgical.)

multiple instruments and telescope to pass through one abdominal incision, which may have some advantages such as minimizing the risk of portal entry complications. The nearness of instruments and telescope may propagate clashing and challenges with triangulation. Success using single-incision access has been well established for procedures such as gonadectomy, gastropexy, and organ biopsy. However, controlled trials investigating such devices are uncommon and advantages over multi-port systems may be difficult to prove.[8]

Successful use of single-incision devices is possible with adequate working space, procedure modification (utility of wound retractor devices), and articulated instruments. Additionally, the safety of resterilization and use of the single incision laparoscopic surgery (SILS) port device (Medtronic, Covidien, Minneapolis, MN) for up to 4 cycles has been established. Alterations to the SILS device after resterilization (loss of flexibility, maneuverability, mechanical damage) may, however, warrant device replacement prior to 4 cycles.[9,10] Recently, progressive utility of the SILS port included modified single-port cisterna chyli ablation with a radial retractor and SILS device in combination.[11] Single-port retroperitoneoscopic adrenalectomy has also been performed in normal dogs.[12] The authors reported feasibility using the SILS device as well as reasonable operative times (mean 44 ± 6.1 minutes). The flexibility of the SILS port appeared to allow for reasonable maneuverability with standard rigid instrumentation, although this procedure has yet to translate to clinical cases. Furthermore, foreign body retrieval in dogs using single-port systems has recently been compared to open laparotomy and found to have similar outcomes, with a moderate risk of conversion (23%).[13]

Transanal access platforms have been evaluated in canine cadaveric models. The SILS port appeared to offer a less personnel- and equipment-demanding alternative to traditional colonoscopy and was feasible in a small cadaveric cohort.[14] Transanal submucosal resection of the canine rectal wall has also been evaluated using Gel-POINT path transanal access platform (CNB10; Applied Medical, Rancho Santa Margarita, CA). Feasibility of distal colonic resections was determined, although the large size of the device was challenging even in large-breed cadavers (median 44.3 kg, range 37.5–60; **Fig. 2**).[15] Clinical translation of these techniques has yet to be explored, to the knowledge of the author.

In addition to the purpose-made single-incision devices, a glove port system has been described as an economic alternative to conventional single-incision port systems. The early experience with this device in human hospitals was first published in 2010[16,17] and combined a radial ring retractor, sterile glove, and standard laparoscopic trocars into a functional single-incision device. Recently, this device was used for laparoscopic ovariohysterectomy (OVH) in dogs,[18] with comparable surgical times (median 24 minutes, range 17.5–39.5) and complication rates to standard laparoscopic OVH. The assembly time of the device varied but appeared to shorten in the latter half of the study suggesting a learning curve. Prior to this, a single report of the surgical glove port for a laparoscopic-assisted OVH for pyometra was described.[19]

Performance of the SILS device has also been compared to the surgical glove port in a novice simulator model for simple tasks (peg transfer and pattern cutting), with the glove port outperforming the SILS port in both tasks. Interestingly, the glove port showed improved maneuverability compared to the SILS port. While there is limited translation to clinical cases performed by laparoscopic surgeons, this suggests potential comparable utility to the SILS as well as potential advantages (maneuverability at the port body wall interface).[20] The use of the glove port for laparoscopic OVH or ovariectomy, and potentially other procedures, appears safe and reasonable.

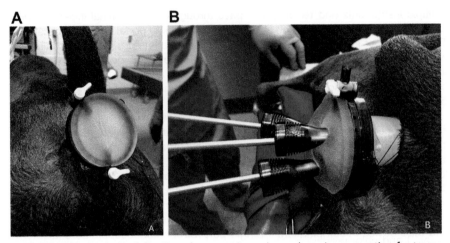

Fig. 2. (A) GelPoint device following placement in canine cadaver in preparation for transanal biopsy acquisition; GelSeal cap (center) placed onto GelSeal sheath. (B) GelSeal device following placement in canine cadaver with cannulas and subsequent instruments in preparation for transanal biopsy acquisition. (*Courtesy of* Philipp D. Mayhew, BVM&S, DACVS-SA, Davis, CA.)

MULTIPORT CANNULA SYSTEMS

While multiport systems remain much the same in veterinary medicine, there is increasing interest in improving smoke evacuation, pneumoperitoneum management, and surgical vision optimization. Surgical smoke generated from electrosurgical instruments is considered an occupational safety hazard, and smoke evacuation systems have been recommended or required. High concentration of harmful volatile organic compounds in the operating room was demonstrated in both MIS and open procedures, with comparable means although generally higher maximum concentrations within the open procedure cohort. Importantly, smoke evacuation systems were found to effectively lower maximum concentrations of certain harmful substances, supporting their use.[21] A novel valveless trocar (AirSeal, ConMed, Largo, FL) contains a filtered circulatory flow design which enables simultaneous insufflation and pressure sensing as well as constant smoke evacuation, also leading to less camera fogging.[22,23] This is at odds to standard insufflators, which alternate pressure sensing and insufflation. Some benefits of this novel trocar technology include reduced CO_2 gas consumption and absorption, which may be beneficial in patients with reduced cardiopulmonary function.[23] In robotic prostatectomies, fewer episodes of pressure loss,[24] as well as shorter operative times, less pain intensity within the first 18 hours, and less nausea, were reported in the valveless trocar group compared to standard trocars.[25] Information regarding this device in veterinary surgery is lacking, although similar translation of benefits may be expected. The pliant abdomen of cats and small dogs may especially benefit from mitigation of pneumoperitoneum loss. Procedures such as laparoscopic adrenalectomy, which frequently rely on suctioning, may benefit from sustained pressure sensing/insufflation as well.

Commercial or homemade smoke evacuation devices for laparoscopy suggested by the European Association for Endoscopic Surgery,[26] SeeClear MAX (Cooper Surgical, Trumbull, CT), S-PILOT (Karl Storz, 78532 Tuttlingen, Germany) among others, may provide similar advantages, although additional research is required.

ANTILENS FOGGING TECHNOLOGY

Lens fogging has plagued MIS and inspired substantial mitigation efforts. Lens fogging can impair vision, increase operative time, and may contribute to intraoperative complications. Generation of lens fog is considered to be the imbalance of cold lens temperature and warm humidity of the abdominal cavity.[27,28] In addition to the valveless trocars (described earlier), warming devices and various solutions have been developed and evaluated. The author has considerable experience with the topical surfactant Fred (Covidien, Dublin, Ireland), although other solutions such as ResoClear (Resorba, Nuremberg, Germany) or Ultra-Stop (Sigmapharm, Vienna, Austria) exist as well. The performance of various antifog techniques in simulation trials has shown conflicting results. Recently, Fred outperformed scope warmers, Betadine, chlorhexidine, and ResoClear solutions,[27] under simulated lens fogging conditions. Conversely, in a similar simulation trial, warmed saline and chlorhexidine solution performed better than Fred.[29] In the clinical setting, warmed saline protected better against fog generation than antifog solutions (Ultra-Stop,[30] ResoClear[28]) and chlorhexidine.[30] While there appears to be some discrepancy in the literature, a recent systematic review regarding antifog techniques concluded that heated sterile water, heated laparoscope lenses, and surfactant solutions were more effective than other alternatives at minimizing lens fog. However, clinically important outcomes (operative times, complications, length of stay) were not associated with any device/technique.[31] While veterinary studies are lacking, it may be prudent for veterinary surgeons to consider warmed sterile water or saline if cost-restricted, although surfactant solutions may be equally effective in reducing lens fog.

IMAGE ACQUISITION: 3 DIMENSIONAL, 4K ULTRAHIGH-DEFINITION, AND WIDE-VIEW LAPAROSCOPY TECHNOLOGY

Three-dimensional (3D) technology has been investigated for the improvement in depth perception. Standard laparoscopy leads to the reduction of depth perception, which may lead to the misjudgment of objects and their positions relative to the surgeons' instruments and each other. In 2D, monoscopic visual cues such as overlap, texture, and size familiarity remain for the surgeon to partially reconstruct a 3D view, which is much reduced compared to the typical binocular view. Stereopsis, leading to the perception of depth, is essential in surgery. Inability to accurately move through the surgical field may lead to complications that have real ramifications for patients undergoing MIS.[32]

3D video monitors have been introduced in human and veterinary surgery, although there remains hesitancy to adopt 3D imaging due to perceived or real side effects such as visual strain, headache, nausea, and tiredness, which appear to be most important if the 3D device is inappropriately set up.[33–37]

In veterinary medicine, a single case report utilizing 3D imaging and a prospective randomized controlled trial (RCT) of 3D compared to 2D imaging for laparoscopic gastropexy are available.[38,39] In the latter report, laparoscopic gastropexy was not shorter, or easier according to NASA-task load index (TLX) surgeon workload index, with 3D imaging compared to 2D imaging. Mixed results have been reported also in human medicine, with an appreciable dearth of information in the clinical utility of 3D imaging. The European Academy of Endoscopy Surgeons reviewed evidence associated with utility of 3D imaging, finding reasonable level of evidence of reduction in operative time, but less strong consensus regarding rate of complications. Complicated tasks such as suturing may gain some advantage with 3D imaging. Fewer gallbladder perforations occurred and critical dissection time in the triangle of Calot was reduced with 3D for complex cholecystectomy patients in one randomized controlled trial, although overall error frequency and operative times were not different.[36] Similarly, 3D guidance improved certain anatomical plane excisions for rectal cancer while overall performance, surgeon workload, and perioperative outcomes were not different in 2D versus 3D.[35] A gastric cancer RCT demonstrated less intraoperative blood loss in the 3D group compared to the 2D group while there was no difference between operative times.[34] While a complete review of the clinical utility of 3D is beyond the scope of this article, it appears that subtle advantages to the stereopsis provided by 3D imaging may lead to some advantages in specific procedures, and there is some consensus on advantages pertaining to operative times and complication rates. The clinical ramifications of these may be difficult to elucidate in veterinary patients, and so applying the evidence that exists in human literature to small animal patients should be considered.

Regarding nonclinical training scenarios, a recent meta-analysis identified no difference in performance of clinical cases (hysterectomy), while errors on standardized tasks (peg transfer, cutting, suturing) were significantly reduced with 3D versus 2D vision.[40] Similarly, the European Association of Endoscopic Surgeons identified improved task performance in the box trainer arena with 3D cameras, although translation of box trainer performance of basic tasks to clinical performance has yet to be gleaned.[37]

Ultra high-definition (HD) endovision systems (4K or 8K) are another method of minimizing the limitations inherent to 2D vision in the surgical field. Sharpening the image quality may allow better identification of landmarks and vascular structures. The advanced image resolution resulting from 4 times the pixels compared to standard high definition has led to improved detail and ability to zoom/magnify the image. While 4K imaging performance compared to 3D may be secondary in a box trainer setting,[41] it continues to be considered standard of care in the clinical setting. The higher resolution of 4K ultra HD video is intended to improve depth perception, dissection precision, and hemostasis, and compared to standard vision, 4K technology may provide objective benefit in reducing intraoperative blood loss and operative time.[42] Specific clinical evaluation of this technology and comparison to 3D vision is limited in the clinical setting, although it seems that the use of 4K technology in laparoscopy and thoracoscopy is valuable and a reasonable alternative to 3D imaging.

Newer expanded field-of-view (FOV) laparoscopes have recently been investigated. Potential advantages of this novel laparoscope include improved instrument viewing, mitigation of vision loss from smoke or fog, and subsequent improvement to the flow of surgery.[43] SurroundScope (270Surgical, Natanya, Israel) is a novel wide-angled laparoscope with a central image sensor covering 95° to 115° of view with side sensors that can extend the FOV to 270°. This device was found to be safe and tolerable by the surgeon, and smoke and fog was not found to interfere with the procedure.[43] It was suggested that the improved ability to map and view port sites and instruments with a wider view may mitigate various possible surgical complications. Subsequently, the expanded FOV laparoscope was found to improve workflow in laparoscopic cholecystectomies compared to standard laparoscopes by decreasing entries into the FOV, identifying instruments and ports more often, with fewer removals to manage fog/smoke compared to standard cameras.[44] Compared to standard laparoscopes, there was shorter trocar duration, time to critical view of safety, and operative duration in the group with enhanced FOV.[45] Availability and application of this technology in human and veterinary MIS continues to be an interesting future endeavor.

HEMOSTATIC DEVICES: STAPLERS, BIPOLAR AND ULTRASONIC VESSEL-SEALING DEVICES, AND PRETIED LIGATURE LOOPS

Endoscopic staple devices have remained essential in minimally invasive hilar transections in small animals, especially in hilar lung lobectomy. Graduated compression staplers, employed by Tri-Staple (Medtronic, Minneapolis, MN) is a novel technology that uses 6 rows of staples, with progressively smaller staple size as the rows approach the line of transection. The idea behind the technology is to apply less stress on the tissues engaged within the staples and improve perfusion to the staple edge,[46] although these advantages remain unclear in thoracoscopic pulmonary surgery. Two sizes of tri-staple cartridge technology were compared to standard staples (EndoGIA, Medtronic, Minneapolis, MN) for lung biopsy in a canine cadaveric study and leak pressures and were significantly lower with the tri-staple technology-acquired lung biopsy compared to standard staples (mean 29.2 and 26 cmH_2O compared to 38 cmH_2O). This is suggestive that the tri-staple technology may be inadequate for peripheral lung biopsy in some cases.[47] Historical data regarding thoracoscopic hilar lung lobectomy in dogs support the successful use of the Endo-GIA standard stapler, but incomplete sectioning of the hilus requiring multiple cartridges remains the primary issues with this device.[48,49] Further research is necessary to elucidate the role and function of tri-staple technology in thoracoscopy in small animals.

Vessel-sealing technologies, including the LigaSure (Medtronic, Minneapolis, MN), SurgRX EnSeal device (Ethicon, Cincinnati, PH), and the ultrasonic energy technology of the Harmonic system (Ethicon Endo-surgery, Raritan, NJ), have been relied upon for their convenience regarding sealing, transection, and dissecting in general thoracoscopic and laparoscopic surgery. These devices have been well evaluated for important outcome parameters such as vessel diameter, burst strength, and thermal spread. Resterilization and device reusability is essential when weighing cost-sensitivity of veterinary medicine with device function and ultimately patient safety. A recent study compared the performance of the LigaSure 5 mm blunt tip, Caiman (Braun Vetcare, 78532 Tuttlingen, Germany) 5 mm tip, and the novel reusable MarSeal 5 plus (KLS Martin, 78532 Tuttlingen, Germany). There was no correlation between burst pressure and seals (totaling 25 per device), and all devices functioned throughout 5 sterilization cycles with the exception of a single Caiman device following the fourth sterilization cycle.[50] Furthermore, 5 mm LigaSure Maryland devices underwent repeated sterilization cycles until failure, which ranged from 4 to 12 cycles with a mean $\pm$ SD of 7.7 $\pm$ 2.8.[51] This suggests that limited reuse of these devices is reasonable and safe. Additional risk regarding electrosurgical devices in thoracoscopy has been recently suggested with the rare, but often malignant ventricular fibrillation in dogs undergoing pericardiectomy.[52] The cautious association between the use of monopolar and bipolar electrosurgery devices and ventricular arrhythmia during pericardiectomy should lead to careful and even limited use of these devices during pericardiectomy.

A new promising device evaluated in cadaveric lung biopsy is the Caiman vessel-sealing device, which is able to seal vessels up to 7 mm with thermal spread of less than 1 mm. The longer jaw tips (26.5 mm for 5 mm hand piece and 50 mm for 12 mm hand piece) enable larger sealing surface and have a "tip first" closure that prevents tissue slippage from the jaws and enables more even pressure distribution compared to the LigaSure device.[53] The suggested benefit of even pressure distribution within the jaws is a more homogenous quality of seal. Burst pressures exceeded 300 mm Hg independent of outer diameter of vessel in experimental vascular canine and porcine models. Additionally, there is 80° jaw articulation, enabling improved dexterity.[53] Peripheral lung biopsy and total lung lobectomy were evaluated on 12 lung lobes in cadaveric specimens (32 and 65 kg). Mean leak pressures for the lung biopsy group were 39.17 ± 13.2 cm H_2O and 38.33 ± 13.67 cm H_2O for total lung lobectomy; thermal damage extended 2.7 ± 0.1 mm. In the largest specimen, none of the total lung lobectomies leaked at less than 20 mm Hg, which suggests some clinical utility.[54] A single case report describes successful video assisted thoracoscopic surgery (VATS) partial lung lobectomy with the Caiman to treat a bulla in the right middle lung lobe of a Shih Tzu.[55] More robust clinical reports of this devices' utility in thoracoscopic procedures is required, although the potential advantages of this device over the more routinely used vessel sealing equipment may benefit laparoscopic or thoracoscopic use.

The harmonic ultrasonic vessel-sealing device controls bleeding through denaturing of protein secondary to blade vibrations leading to a coagulum formation sealing small vessels; prolonged effects include heat and sealing of larger vessels.[56] The advantages of the harmonic device over other vessel-sealing devices include minimized thermal spread.[56] Utility of the harmonic scalpel in small animal MIS is not well described, although the successful use reported for two feline laparoscopic adrenalectomycases is encouraging.[57] Successful use has also been documented in canine laparoscopic adrenalectomy in dogs (along with other bipolar and ultrasonic vessel-sealing devices), although how this, and other devices, related to patient outcomes was not directly evaluated.[58] Ultimately, it remains unclear whether there is any bipolar or ultrasonic vessel-sealing device that outperforms the other in a clinical setting, and continued experience with old and newer technologies will allow ongoing evaluation.

Pretied ligature loops (PLLs) are suture loops passed through a long thin plastic tube, circumferentially scored where the suture attaches. The scored end is snapped and pulled when the loop is positioned around the pedicle of interest, and pretied loop secured. This device has been evaluated in cadaveric lung lobes for performance in lung lobe biopsy 3 cm away from the lung lobe edge. Cadaveric lung lobes that were biopsied with a ligature loop (Surgitie ligating loop, Medtronic, Minneapolis, MIN) sustained pressures up to a median of 40 cmH_2O, failing at 30 cmH_2O in one sample of 2-0, while remaining samples (2-0 and 0) sustained pressures of up to 40 cmH_2O. This was favorable when compared to other techniques (vessel-sealing device, endo-GIA 45 stapler, square knot, or modified 4S Roeder knot)[59]; the PLL has since been evaluated in cadaveric models and clinical cases of open (4 dogs) or thoracoscopic-assisted (1 dog) lung lobectomy with success. Importantly, of the 5 clinical cases reported, all clinical cases had sustained, reliable seals.[60] The translation of PLL to thoracoscopic lung lobectomy, including technical feasibility, remains necessary.

SUMMARY

New technology is in constant development to enable growth of MIS. Suitability of novel devices to veterinary medicine, and veterinary patients, while acknowledging limitations (resources, finances) inherent to many veterinary practices, requires careful interpretation of technology in human medicine. While there is some veterinary focused literature discussing novel technologies, the translation of human-focused literature should be considered.

CLINICS CARE POINTS

- Reusability and resterilization of vessel-sealing devices appears to be safe, although limiting cycles to ensure that function is maintained and the risk of contamination is minimized is prudent.
- Optimizing surgical views in laparoscopy and thoracoscopy is key to success and flow of surgery
  - There does not appear to be consistent superiority of antifog devices.
  - Three-dimensional technology may allow for improved performance in certain procedures or portions of procedures (such as intracorporeal suturing) in which stereopsis is key, and further investigation into clinical utility is indicated.
  - Wide-view laparoscopy may optimize surgical flow, patient safety, and surgical success and should be considered for translation into veterinary minimally invasive surgery.
  - Valveless trocar technology may allow for sustained pneumoperitoneum and clearer surgical view.
- Articulating nonmechanized instrumentation may suit the growing need for improved intraoperative dexterity to match the increasingly advanced minimally invasive procedures that are performed in veterinary medicine.
- Smoke evacuation systems are indicated for laparoscopic surgery to optimize surgeon and/or staff safety. Various systems are available, although further studies are required to establish superiority.
- Various hemostatic devices such as ultrasonic and bipolar vessel-sealing devices, staplers, and pretied ligature loops are available to veterinary minimally invasive surgeons
  - Tri-staple technology may not be optimally suited for lung biopsy, although appear to function well for hilar lung lobectomies.
  - Utility and success of various hemostatic and ligating devices may vary based on the size and type of tissue operated, and familiarity with strengths and weaknesses of specific devices is recommended prior to use in minimally invasive surgery.

DISCLOSURE

The author has no disclosures to declare.

REFERENCES

1. Awtar S, Trutna TT, Nielsen JM, et al. FlexDex™: A Minimally Invasive Surgical Tool With Enhanced Dexterity and Intuitive Control. J Med Devices 2010;4:035003.
2. Lee E, Lee K, Kang SH, et al. Usefulness of articulating laparoscopic instruments during laparoscopic gastrectomy for gastric adenocarcinoma. J Minim Invasive Surg 2021;24(1):35–42.
3. Kang SH, Hwang D, Yoo M, et al. Feasibility of articulating laparoscopic instruments in laparoscopic gastrectomy using propensity score matching. Sci Rep 2023;13(1):17384.
4. Min SH, Cho YS, Park K, et al. Multi-DOF (Degree of Freedom) Articulating Laparoscopic Instrument is an Effective Device in Performing Challenging Sutures. J Minim Invasive Surg 2019;22(4):157–63.
5. Lee CM, Park S, Park SH, et al. Short-term outcomes and cost-effectiveness of laparoscopic gastrectomy with articulating instruments for gastric cancer compared with the robotic approach. Sci Rep 2023;13:9355.
6. Criss CN, Jarboe MD, Claflin J, et al. Evaluating a Solely Mechanical Articulating Laparoscopic Device: A Prospective Randomized Crossover Study. J Laparoendosc Adv Surg Tech 2019;29(4):542–50.

7. Motahariasl N, Farzaneh SB, Motahariasl S, et al. Assessment of an Articulating Laparoscopic Needle Holder (FlexDex™) Compared to a Conventional Rigid Needle Holder in 2-Dimension Vision Amongst Novices: A Randomised Controlled Study. Med Devices Auckl NZ 2022;15:15–25.

8. Lacitignola L, Guadalupi M, Massari F. Single Incision Laparoscopic Surgery (SILS) in Small Animals: A Systematic Review and Meta-Analysis of Current Veterinary Literature. Vet Sci 2021;8(8):144.

9. Petrovsky B, Monnet E. Evaluation of efficacy of repeated decontamination and sterilization of single-incision laparoscopic surgery ports intended for 1-time use. Vet Surg 2018;47(S1):O52–8.

10. Coisman JG, Case JB, Clark ND, et al. Efficacy of decontamination and sterilization of a single-use single-incision laparoscopic surgery port. Am J Vet Res 2013; 74(6):934–8.

11. Morris KP, Singh A, Holt DE, et al. Hybrid single-port laparoscopic cisterna chyli ablation for the adjunct treatment of chylothorax disease in dogs. Vet Surg 2019; 48(S1):O121–9.

12. Ko J, Jeong J, Lee S, et al. Feasibility of single-port retroperitoneoscopic adrenalectomy in dogs. Vet Surg 2018;47(Suppl 1):O75–83.

13. Otomo A, Singh A, Valverde A, et al. Comparison of outcome in dogs undergoing single-incision laparoscopic-assisted intestinal surgery and open laparotomy for simple small intestinal foreign body removal. Vet Surg 2019;48(S1):O83–90.

14. Howard J, Bertran J, Parker V, et al. Transanal access port (TrAAP) technique: the use of a single incision laparoscopic surgical port during canine colonoscopy (a cadaveric study). BMC Vet Res 2021;17(1):43.

15. Mayhew PD, Balsa IM, Guerzon CN, et al. Evaluation of transanal minimally invasive surgery for submucosal rectal resection in cadaveric canine specimens. Vet Surg 2020;49(7):1378–87.

16. Jeon HG, Jeong W, Oh CK, et al. Initial Experience With 50 Laparoendoscopic Single Site Surgeries Using a Homemade, Single Port Device at a Single Center. J Urol 2010;183(5):1866–72.

17. Tai HC, Lin CD, Wu CC, et al. Homemade transumbilical port: an alternative access for laparoendoscopic single-site surgery (LESS). Surg Endosc 2010;24(3): 705–8.

18. Bydzovsky ND, Bockstahler B, Dupré G. Single-port laparoscopic-assisted ovariohysterectomy with a modified glove-port technique in dogs. Vet Surg 2019; 48(5):715–25.

19. Becher-Deichsel A, Aurich JE, Schrammel N, et al. A surgical glove port technique for laparoscopic-assisted ovariohysterectomy for pyometra in the bitch. Theriogenology 2016;86(2):619–25.

20. Strohmeier U, Dupré G, Bockstahler B, et al. Comparison of a single-access glove port with a SILS™ port in a surgical simulator model using MISTELS. BMC Vet Res 2021;17(1):285.

21. Kocher GJ, Koss AR, Groessl M, et al. Electrocautery smoke exposure and efficacy of smoke evacuation systems in minimally invasive and open surgery: a prospective randomized study. Sci Rep 2022;12(1):4941.

22. Bracale U, Silvestri V, Pontecorvi E, et al. Smoke Evacuation During Laparoscopic Surgery: A Problem Beyond the COVID-19 Period. A Quantitative Analysis of CO_2 Environmental Dispersion Using Different Devices. Surg Innov 2022;29(2):154–9.

23. Herati AS, Andonian S, Rais-Bahrami S, et al. Use of the Valveless Trocar System Reduces Carbon Dioxide Absorption During Laparoscopy When Compared With Standard Trocars. Urology 2011;77(5):1126–32.

24. Horstmann M, Horton K, Kurz M, et al. Prospective comparison between the Air-Seal® System valve-less Trocar and a standard Versaport™ Plus V2 Trocar in robotic-assisted radical prostatectomy. J Endourol 2013;27(5):579–82.

25. Shahait M, Cockrell R, Yezdani M, et al. Improved Outcomes Utilizing a Valveless-Trocar System during Robot-assisted Radical Prostatectomy (RARP). J Soc Laparoendosc Surg 2019;23(1). e2018.00085.

26. Mintz Y, Arezzo A, Boni L, et al. A Low-cost, Safe, and Effective Method for Smoke Evacuation in Laparoscopic Surgery for Suspected Coronavirus Patients. Ann Surg 2020;272(1):e7.

27. Manning TG, Papa N, Perera M, et al. Laparoscopic lens fogging: solving a common surgical problem in standard and robotic laparoscopes via a scientific model. Surg Endosc 2018;32(3):1600–6.

28. Merkx R, Muselaers C, d'Ancona F, et al. Effectiveness of Heated Sterile Water vs ResoClear® for Prevention of Laparoscopic Lens Fogging in a Randomized Comparative Trial. J Endourol 2018;32(1):54–8.

29. Palvia V, Gonzalez AJH, Vigh RS, et al. A Randomized Controlled Trial Comparing Laparoscopic Lens Defogging Techniques through Simulation Model. Gynecol Minim Invasive Ther 2018;7(4):156–60.

30. Song T, Lee DH. A randomized Comparison of laparoscopic LEns defogging using Anti-fog solution, waRm saline, and chlorhexidine solution (CLEAR). Surg Endosc 2020;34(2):940–5.

31. Nabeel A, Al-Sabah SK, Ashrafian H. Effective cleaning of endoscopic lenses to achieve visual clarity for minimally invasive abdominopelvic surgery: a systematic review. Surg Endosc 2022;36(4):2382–92.

32. Bogdanova R, Boulanger P, Zheng B. Depth Perception of Surgeons in Minimally Invasive Surgery. Surg Innov 2016;23(5):515–24.

33. Mueller MD, Camartin C, Dreher E, et al. Three-dimensional laparoscopy. Surg Endosc 1999;13(5):469–72.

34. Zheng CH, Lu J, Zheng HL, et al. Comparison of 3D laparoscopic gastrectomy with a 2D procedure for gastric cancer: A phase 3 randomized controlled trial. Surgery 2018;163(2):300–4.

35. Curtis NJ, Conti JA, Dalton R, et al. 2D versus 3D laparoscopic total mesorectal excision: a developmental multicentre randomised controlled trial. Surg Endosc 2019;33(10):3370–83.

36. Schwab KE, Curtis NJ, Whyte MB, et al. 3D laparoscopy does not reduce operative duration or errors in day-case laparoscopic cholecystectomy: a randomised controlled trial. Surg Endosc 2020;34(4):1745–53.

37. Arezzo A, Vettoretto N, Francis NK, et al. The use of 3D laparoscopic imaging systems in surgery: EAES consensus development conference 2018. Surg Endosc 2019;33(10):3251–74.

38. Griffin MA, Balsa IM, Mayhew PD. Bilateral intracorporeally sutured inguinal herniorrhaphy using 3-dimensional laparoscopy in a dog. Can Vet J 2021;62(6):572–6.

39. Balsa IM, Giuffrida MA, Mayhew PD. A randomized controlled trial of three-dimensional versus two-dimensional imaging system on duration of surgery and mental workload for laparoscopic gastropexies in dogs. Vet Surg 2021;50(5):944–53.

40. Restaino S, Scutiero G, Taliento C, et al. Three-dimensional vision versus two-dimensional vision on laparoscopic performance of trainee surgeons: a systematic review and meta-analysis. Updat Surg 2023;75(3):455–70.

41. Wahba R, Datta R, Bußhoff J, et al. 3D Versus 4K Display System – Influence of "State-of-the-art"-Display Technique on Surgical Performance (IDOSP-study) in Minimally Invasive Surgery. Ann Surg 2020;272(5):709–14.

42. Mari GM, Crippa J, Achilli P, et al. 4K ultra HD technology reduces operative time and intraoperative blood loss in colorectal laparoscopic surgery. F1000Research 2020;9:106.

43. Thompson KJ, Sroka G, Loveitt AP, et al. The introduction of wide-angle 270° laparoscopy through a novel laparoscopic camera system. Surg Endosc 2022;36(3): 2151–8.

44. Ehrlich Z, Shapira SS, Sroka G. Effects of wide-angle laparoscopy on surgical workflow in laparoscopic cholecystectomies. Surg Endosc 2023;37(7):5760–5.

45. Shapira SS, Ehrlich Z, Koren P, et al. Comparing a novel wide field of view laparoscope with conventional laparoscope while performing laparoscopic cholecystectomy. Surg Endosc 2023. https://doi.org/10.1007/s00464-023-10393-3.

46. Eschbach M, Sindberg GM, Godek ML, et al. Micro-CT imaging as a method for comparing perfusion in graduated-height and single-height surgical staple lines. Med Devices Auckl NZ 2018;11:267–73.

47. Imhoff DJ, Monnet E. Inflation Pressures for Ex Vivo Lung Biopsies After Application of Graduated Compression Staples. Vet Surg VS 2016;45(1):79–82.

48. Mayhew PD, Hunt GB, Steffey MA, et al. Evaluation of short-term outcome after lung lobectomy for resection of primary lung tumors via video-assisted thoracoscopic surgery or open thoracotomy in medium- to large-breed dogs. J Am Vet Med Assoc 2013;243(5):681–8.

49. Lansdowne JL, Monnet E, Twedt DC, et al. Thoracoscopic Lung Lobectomy for Treatment of Lung Tumors in Dogs. Vet Surg 2005;34(5):530–5.

50. Gardeweg S, Bockstahler B, Duprè G. Effect of multiple use and sterilization on sealing performance of bipolar vessel sealing devices. PLoS One 2019;14(8): e0221488.

51. Valenzano D, Hayes G, Gludish D, et al. Performance and microbiological safety testing after multiple use cycles and hydrogen peroxide sterilization of a 5-mm vessel-sealing device. Vet Surg 2019;48(5):885–9.

52. Raleigh JS, Mayhew PD, Visser LC, et al. The development of ventricular fibrillation as a complication of pericardiectomy in 16 dogs. Vet Surg 2022;51(4): 611–9.

53. Eick S, Loudermilk B, Walberg E, et al. Rationale, bench testing and in vivo evaluation of a novel 5 mm laparoscopic vessel sealing device with homogeneous pressure distribution in long instrument jaws. Ann Surg Innov Res 2013; 7(1):15.

54. Brückner M, Heblinski N, Henrich M. Use of a novel vessel-sealing device for peripheral lung biopsy and lung lobectomy in a cadaveric model. J Small Anim Pract 2019;60(7):411–6.

55. Zobe A, Rohwedder T, Böttcher P. Partial lung lobectomy with the Caiman® Seal & Cut device in a dog with spontaneous pneumothorax: Case report. Open Vet J 2022;12(6):910–8.

56. Noble EJ, Smart NJ, Challand C, et al. Experimental comparison of mesenteric vessel sealing and thermal damage between one bipolar and two ultrasonic shears devices. Br J Surg 2011;98(6):797–800.

57. Zhang RM, Case JB. Use of a Harmonic scalpel for laparoscopic adrenalectomy in two cats. J Feline Med Surg Open Rep 2023;9(1). 20551169231159635.

58. Mayhew PD, Massari F, Araya FL, et al. Laparoscopic adrenalectomy for resection of unilateral noninvasive adrenal masses in dogs is associated with excellent outcomes in experienced centers. J Am Vet Med Assoc 2023;1(aop):1–8.
59. Marvel S, Monnet E. Ex Vivo Evaluation of Canine Lung Biopsy Techniques. Vet Surg 2013;42(4):473–7.
60. Cronin AM, Pustelnik SB, Owen L, et al. Evaluation of a pre-tied ligature loop for canine total lung lobectomy. Vet Surg 2019;48(4):570–7.

Looking to the Future; Veterinary Robotic Surgery

Nicole J. Buote, DVM, DACVS

KEYWORDS

- Robotics • Robotic surgery • Da Vinci • EndoWrist • Robotic gastropexy
- Psychomotor skills

KEY POINTS

- Surgical robots have been used since the early 1990's for a variety of surgical procedures including urogenital, orthopedic, and gynecologic.
- Surgical robots have 3 main components (patient side cart, vision cart, and surgeon console) that work together to allow for the primary surgeon to control the robotic arms and instrumentation away from the patient table.
- The main advantage to robotic surgery is the articulated instrumentation which allows for precise dissection and suturing in small hard to reach spaces.
- Robotic procedures have been successfully performed on live veterinary patients for prophylactic and corrective therapies, and continued work is ongoing.

 Video content accompanies this article at http://www.vetsmall.theclinics.com.

HISTORY OF SURGICAL ROBOTICS

The history of surgical robotics is a testament to human ingenuity, innovation, and the relentless pursuit of precision in medicine. Surgical robotics emerged as a concept in the late 20th century, inspired by the desire to overcome the limitations of traditional surgery. The realization of this dream can be attributed to a handful of pioneering individuals and the convergence of several technological advancements. The first pivotal moment in the history of surgical robotics came in 1985 when the PUMA 560, a robotic arm developed by Victor Scheinman of the Unimation company, was used for neurosurgical procedures.[1,2] This system, also known as the Program for Universal Machine Assembly 560, was a widely used industrial robot. It was popular due to its versatility and precision in various manufacturing and industrial applications. The robot was known for its 6° of freedom, which allowed it to move and position its end-effector (the peripheral device that attaches to a robot's wrist, allowing the robot to

Minimally Invasive Surgery (Soft Tissue), Cornell University College of Veterinary Medicine, Small Animal Surgery, 930 Campus Road, Ithaca, NY 14853, USA
E-mail address: Njb235@cornell.edu

Vet Clin Small Anim 54 (2024) 735–751
https://doi.org/10.1016/j.cvsm.2024.02.008
0195-5616/24/© 2024 Elsevier Inc. All rights reserved.

interact with its task) with great flexibility. It was controlled by a computer and could be programmed to perform a wide range of tasks in industrial settings. The robotic system not only allowed for precise movements but also stable movements, allowing its crossover into minimally invasive surgery.

In 1992, the ROBODOC system was introduced for orthopedic surgery. Designed by Dr William Bargar and Dr Howard Paul (a veterinarian), this system was instrumental in precisely shaping bones during total hip and knee replacement surgeries.[3] ROBODOC used a combination of robotic arms and computer software to assist surgeons in removing damaged bone and precisely implanting artificial joints. This system was pre-programed before the operation using CT scans to create a 3D model of the affected joint. During surgery, the robot would use this model to assist the surgeon in making precise cuts and to aid in the placement of the implants. The ROBODOC was an early indicator of the potential of robotics in enhancing surgical outcomes as it aimed to improve the precision and accuracy of orthopedic surgeries.[4,5] While the ROBODOC system was considered a technological breakthrough in its time, it faced some challenges, including the complexity of its operation, the time required for setup, and the cost of the system.[6,7] Over time, it became less popular as newer surgical robot systems emerged.

The most iconic and transformative article in the history of surgical robotics began in the late 1990s with the introduction of the da Vinci Surgical System. Developed by Intuitive Surgical, this system revolutionized soft tissue minimally invasive surgery. The da Vinci system features a surgeon console, robotic arms (patient side cart), and a vision cart. An endoscope, which allows for 3D visualization adds to the surgeon's ability to perform precise, intricate movements. The da Vinci system was approved for assisting in surgery in 1997 and for full use in human patients in 2000 by the FDA, and it quickly gained global recognition. The advantages of the da Vinci over previous robotic systems were the articulated instrumentation which allowed for natural hand and wrist movements and the 3D visualization. The da Vinci system has been utilized in various applications including urology, gynecology, cardiology, and general surgery and surgeons have performed procedures on patients located thousands of miles away, pushing the boundaries of what was once considered possible.[8–15]

ADVANTAGES OF ROBOTICS OVER LAPAROSCOPY

The major advantages to robotic surgery include combining the available magnification and illumination of laparoscopy with the versatility of a three-dimensional field of view and enhanced dexterity in instrumentation (**Box 1**). The improved degrees of freedom of 7 versus 5 in traditional laparoscopy dramatically improve the ergonomics

---

Box 1
Advantages of robotic surgery

Improved visualization (3D) for precise dissection

Improved dexterity
   7 degrees of freedom
   Articulation

Simultaneous retraction and dissection due to articulation

Access to tighter anatomic areas (pelvic canal, thoracic inlet, and so forth)

Ergonomics

for surgeons[16,17] The added articulation of the instruments available with the da Vinci robot also allow for their use in tight spaces and for intricate procedures such as suturing.[18,19] Prior to this development, minimally invasive procedures for advanced urologic, gynecologic, and gastrointestinal diseases were limited. While laparoscopy allowed for increased magnification and illumination, retraction, dissection, and suturing were difficult. The design of robotic instrumentation allows for intuitive movements of the surgeon's hands at the console and mimics the wrist movements of open surgery. Multiple studies have illustrated that robotic surgery is more easily adapted to by general surgeons compared with laparoscopy, which relies on straight instrumentation.[18,20,21] In 2014, Kim and colleagues reported improvements in the performance of specific tasks in the robotic group over the laparoscopic group in both laparoscopic novices and experienced surgeons, suggesting that previous minimally invasive training may not be required for robotic surgeons.[22]

Another major advantage of robotic surgery is the ergonomic advantage to the surgeon. Work-related musculoskeletal disorders (WRMD) are common in surgery and minimally invasive surgery has a high occurrence rate due to the unnatural arm/wrist movements and table height requirements for many of these procedures.[23–25] A veterinary survey by Jones in 2020 confirmed an increased risk of experienced pain in surgeons who performed laparoscopic procedures at least once a month.[26] The robotic surgeon console is able to be adjusted for head, shoulder, arm position, and leg and feet position at the beginning of the procedure. Additionally, as the procedure progresses, technology such as the clutch function on the master grips, allows the surgeon to reposition their arms and hands to a more comfortable position without moving the instrument in the patient. The system also has a safety feature that locks instruments in place if the surgeon's head moves out of the console viewer which allows surgeons to take a physical break if needed without compromising the positioning of the instruments. This decreases the physical and possibly the mental workload on the surgeon and surgical assistants.[27–29] A systematic review by Shugaba and colleagues concluded that a reduction in musculoskeletal demand was also associated with a decrease in cognitive load during robotic surgery when compared with laparoscopic surgery.[29] While no similar study exists in veterinary medicine, the effects of WRMD in veterinary surgery should not be discounted; therefore, ongoing research is warranted.

EQUIPMENT

While new surgical robotic platforms exist and are ever evolving, the da Vinci surgical robot stands out as the first commercially successful and most used surgical system to date. Developed by Intuitive Surgical Inc., this robotic system has revolutionized the way surgeons perform complex surgeries. Central to the success of the da Vinci Si and Xi iterations are the articulated instruments and enhanced precision its platform provides.[30] The system is comprised of a surgeon console, patient side cart, and vison cart as well as interchangeable instrumentation and 3D camera system. This technology is commonly described as a master-slave system with the surgical console considered the master and the patient side cart with the robotic arms as the slave.

Surgeon Console

As its name implies, the surgeon console is whereby the surgeon sits and controls the robotic arms during the surgical procedure. This console consists of a 3D high-definition viewer, dual hand-operated master controllers/grips, and various foot pedals (**Fig. 1**, Video 1). Many aspects of this console can be adjusted for the height,

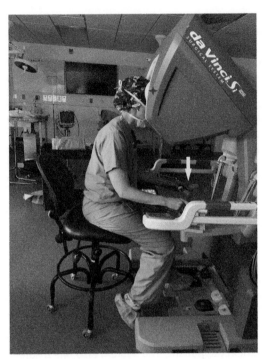

Fig. 1. Photograph of da Vinci Si surgeon console. Yellow arrow denotes the master controllers (or grips). Red star denotes the stereoscopic view finder. (© 2024 Intuitive Surgical Operations, Inc.)

arm length, and the best head and neck positioning for the surgeon. The stereoscopic view at the surgeon console, in addition to the high definition 3D camera, provides a detailed and immersive view of the patient's anatomy with up to 10x magnification. The master controllers or hand grips mimic the surgeon's movements, translating them into precise robotic actions. These controllers also have a clutch function which allows for the instruments to be held steady or locked in place while adjustments to the ergonomics of the hand and arm positioning occur. This is advantageous in many situations. The instruments may be holding delicate tissue or tissue that cannot or should not be regrasped, but the positioning of the surgeon's arms/hands is uncomfortable. By using the clutch function, the surgeon can keep the instruments in place and decrease musculoskeletal strain lessening potential complications. The foot pedals, which can also be adjusted on some models, enable the surgeon to control the camera (focus and position) as well as monopolar and bipolar electrosurgical functions (**Fig. 2**).

Patient Side Cart

The patient side cart contains the robotic arms and is the component that the surgical instruments are attached to before insertion into the body (**Fig. 3**). The da Vinci comes with 3 or 4 arm configurations and one arm is always dedicated to the rigid endoscope and 3D camera assembly. The robotic arms do move around a fixed pivot point but mimic human arm movements and can be equipped with a variety of instruments, which can be easily interchanged during the surgery (Video 2). While autoclavable and reusable, these instruments do have a specified lifespan or number of uses which

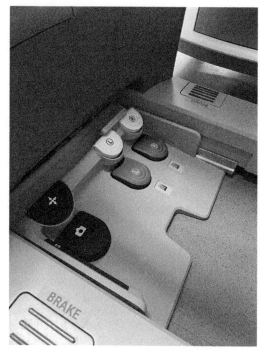

Fig. 2. Photograph of the foot pedals on a da Vinci Si surgeon console. (© 2024 Intuitive Surgical Operations, Inc.)

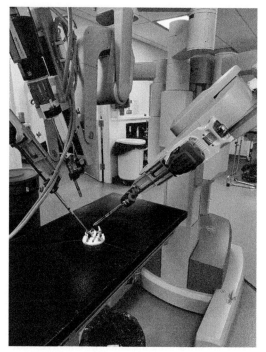

Fig. 3. Photograph of da Vinci Si patient side cart (3-arm). (© 2024 Intuitive Surgical Operations, Inc.)

is tracked by the computer. Port placement is of utmost importance in robotic surgery as the robotic arms must be able to drape over the patient and the arms/instruments will not be able to move toward the main unit (**Fig. 4**).

Vision Cart

The vision cart contains the computer system for the high-definition 3D endoscope, image processing equipment, and widescreen viewing monitor (**Fig. 5**). The monitor is necessary for the patient side assistant to view the progress of the surgical procedure and assist in instrument exchanges. The equipment on the vision cart connects the rigid endoscope and high-definition video to the surgeon console. The image-rendering computers process this visual information and display it on the surgeon's console as a magnified and three-dimensional view of the patient's anatomy. The vision cart can also hold electrosurgical components, stapling devices, and image capture units similar to laparoscopic towers.

EndoWrist Instruments

One of the most important aspects to the da Vinci surgical system's versatility and popularity are the EndoWrist instruments. These instruments are designed with multiple articulating joints near the effector end, enabling them to rotate and bend with a reported 7 degrees of freedom. While only 6 degrees of freedom exist in three-dimensional space (**Fig. 6**), the da Vinci design allows for 7 axes of motions due to the multiple joints of the instrumentation (**Fig. 7**). This is greater than experienced

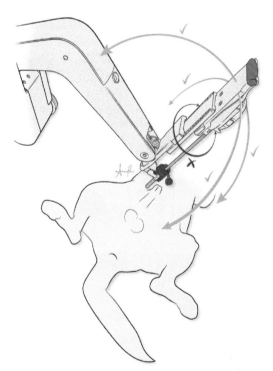

Fig. 4. Illustration of allowable (*green arrows*) and not allowable (*red arrow*) movements for the patient side cart robotic arms. Note the arms/instruments cannot move in a complete circle. Their movements are limited by their attachment to the main unit.

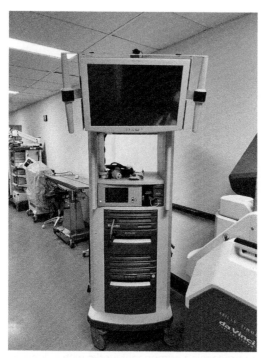

Fig. 5. Photograph of the da Vinci Si Vision cart. (© 2024 Intuitive Surgical Operations, Inc.)

with laparoscopic instruments (5°) and the human wrist (3°) and helps reduce trauma to tissues and surgeon strain during surgery. The EndoWrist instruments come in various diameter sizes (5–12 mm) and types, allowing the surgeon to select the most suitable tool for the task at hand. The enhanced precision the instruments provide allows intricate surgical maneuvers, such as suturing, cutting, and dissecting, to be performed precisely. The articulations of these instruments not only allow for complex maneuvers such as suturing to be completed in tight spaces but also allows for one instrument to be used as a retractor and dissector simultaneously (**Fig. 8**, Video 3). These key features of the robotic system significantly enhance dexterity, when compared with traditional laparoscopy.

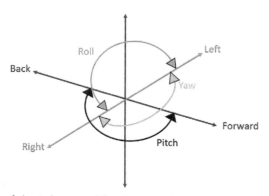

Fig. 6. Illustration of the 6 degrees of freedom in a three-dimensional space.

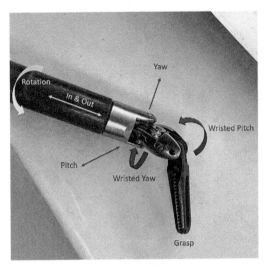

Fig. 7. Labeled photograph of the 7 degrees of freedom possible with articulated robotic instruments.

Firefly Fluorescence Imaging

An additional feature of the da Vinci surgical robot is the Firefly Fluorescence Imaging system. This imaging processing component works with indocyanine green, a fluorophore dye injected to highlight anatomic structures or perfusion. This dye emits

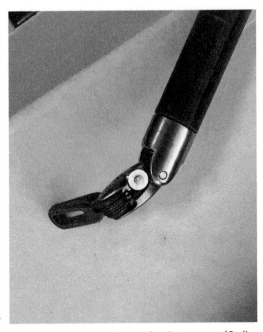

Fig. 8. Photograph of a robotic atraumatic grasping instrument (Cadiere forceps). Note the double articulating at the effector end.

fluorescence (light) at a near-infrared wavelength, with peak emission at 830 nm. The Firefly imaging system provides an external energy (near-infrared light) for indocyanine green to absorb, resulting in the excitation of indocyanine green molecules. The emitted fluorescence is transferred from the field of view to the monitor and processed in real time. This technology is particularly useful in procedures where the precise identification of critical structures is essential, and is usd routinely in biliary, gynecologic, and oncologic surgeries in human medicine.

ROBOTIC PROCEDURES: HUMAN APPLICATIONS

Robotics have been incorporated into all aspects of surgery in human medicine including oncologic, urologic, gynecologic, ophthalmic, neurologic, pediatric, and orthopedic. As data is collected, not every procedure attempted with surgical robots illustrate benefits to patients. The cost of robotic procedures and the length of surgical time must always be balanced with the advantages this advanced equipment may provide.[31] The benefits to patients and surgeons are best experienced when the surgery requires exacting precision, delicate dissection in tight spaces, and suturing. In human surgery, these include procedures such as prostatectomy, hysterectomy, and gastrointestinal anastomoses.[32–42] Prostatectomy is the most well-known procedure performed with a da Vinci robot. In this procedure, challenging dissection around the neurovascular bundle supplying the urinary bladder must be performed to decrease the incidence of postoperative incontinence. The benefits of 3D visualization, magnification, and articulating instrumentation are highly prized in the pelvic canal as even in open surgery this is a difficult space to access. Prostatectomy also requires precise suturing of the urethra to the urinary bladder to avoid postoperative urine leakage and the improved ergonomics and degrees of freedom the robot provides encourages its use over laparoscopy as well.[33,34] In gynecologic cases, especially patients suffering from advanced endometriosis, robotic outcomes have also been shown to be superior to laparoscopic and open surgeries. Accurate dissection around ureters, ovaries, and the urethra when removing metastatic endometrial lesions is a cited advantage and patient satisfaction is high.[35–37]

Other abdominal indications in human medicine include gastric bypass, intestinal resections, and hernia repairs.[38–46] The outcomes of hernia repair with robotics depends on the type and location of the hernia. A recent systematic review and meta-analysis on incisional hernia repair showed no difference regarding postoperative complications or recurrence rate when comparing robotic-assisted surgery (RAS) to laparoscopic repair but patients undergoing robotic surgery experienced a significantly shorter hospital stay.[43] Studies are mixed on the use of robotics in paraesophageal and inguinal hernia repair with no repeatable benefit over laparoscopy[44,45] but significant decreases in postoperative complications and length of stay have been seen in a recent review on robotic hiatal hernia repair.[46] The use of robotics in orthopedic and neurologic procedures centers around the technology's ability to perform precision screw placement and osteotomy procedures. Improved accuracy can lead to decreased postoperative complications and improved patient satisfaction. Many robotic arm systems for orthopedics are linked directly to patient-specific imaging which allows the surgeon to customize the procedure. One recent systematic review with meta-analyses on total knee arthroplasty found that RAS had a better knee alignment and function (Oxford knee score)[47] but a second study reported a less favorable knee alignment and longer surgery times.[48] While results continue to be mixed, robotics appear to be increasingly supported as technology continues to improve and costs begin to decrease.

ROBOTIC PROCEDURES: VETERINARY APPLICATIONS

When discussing the applications of robotics for animal patients it is important to note that all robotic procedures had their beginnings in animal models. Many studies on robotic techniques in animals included experimental animal models for prostatic resections, coronary anastomosis, and pneumonectomy.[48–54] Canine cadavers were described as a relevant and effective training model for prostatectomy highlighting the potential use of robotics in this species.[55] The only clinical report to date in a companion animal is of a robotic radical prostatectomy for a canine with prostatic carcinoma.[56] This Bernese Mountain dog had surgery performed by a human physician trained in robotics using a four-arm da Vinci SI robotic system (**Figs. 9** and **10**). Even though a nerve-sparing approach was performed, the patient was unable to urinate for 3 days postoperatively. The patient required multiple episodes of catheterization but was able to urinate normally at day 7 postoperatively. No intraoperative complications were observed, and the surgery time was noted to be 120 minutes. While this case report did not illustrate a survival benefit of robotic surgery it did illustrate that this procedure can be safely performed in the canine patient.

Investigations into the clinical use of robotics in veterinary medicine are underway. The author's research team reported preclinical feasibility using da Vinci Si surgical system for cholecystectomy in a canine experimental model.[57] Cholecystectomy was chosen for this feasibility study because veterinary patients commonly suffer from biliary disease and surgeons are familiar with the surgical options available. This study also described relevant differences in procedural steps and psychomotor skills between a laparoscopic and a robotic cholecystectomy. Multiple procedural steps are different between these 2 minimally invasive procedures including docking the robotic arms to the ports, verifying adequate range of motion to the arms, instrument exchanges, and surgeon console operations (**Box 2**).

One experienced laparoscopic surgeon performed all of the procedures and recorded not only process differences but also the perceived difficulty of these new processes. A robotic cholecystectomy was successfully performed in all of the canine cadavers with one minor complication of a small gallbladder tear noted. The total procedure time was approximately 120 minutes with 20 minutes devoted to port docking. The most difficult part of the robotic procedure noted was docking the robotic arms and verifying an appropriate range of motion so that the arms did not collide during the procedure. Unlike laparoscopy, the instruments cannot move in a complete circle around the port so careful port site and PSC positioning is crucial(**Box 3**).

The author has recently performed robotic gastropexy on a client-owned patient. The procedure was successful and was performed in less time (26 minutes) than historical laparoscopic gastropexies (45 minutes) even with the inclusion of resident

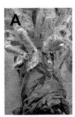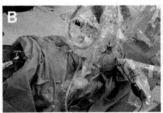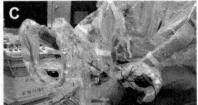

Fig. 9. Positioning of a Bernese mountain dog undergoing robotic prostatectomy with a 4-arm DaVinci SI robotic system. (*A*) view from cranial to caudal, (*B*) right lateral view-patient head to the left of the picture, (*C*) right lateral view with patient's head to the left of the picture and patient in Trendelenburg. (*Courtesy of* Alexander Schlak, DipECVS.)

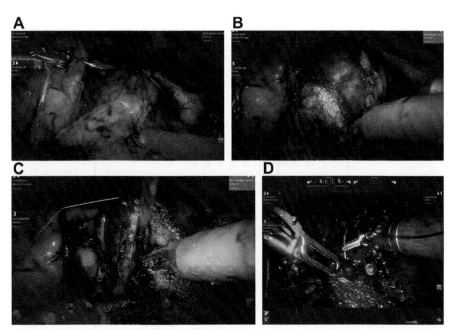

Fig. 10. Intraoperative intracorporeal robotic images during nerve-sparing prostatectomy. (*A*) Identification of the urinary bladder neck, (*B*) dissection of bladder neck from urethra, (*C*) transection of the posterior prostatic urethra, (*D*) anastomosis of urethra to urinary bladder. (*Courtesy of* Alexander Schlak, DipECVS.)

training. The articulated needle holders allowed for the intuitive passing of the needle between hands and suturing of the stomach to the body wall. Ongoing research comparing robotic and laparoscopic techniques are under way with special attention paid to training, ergonomics, and advanced abdominal procedures (hernia repair, anastomoses, and urogenital procedures).

Box 2 **Robotic-specific skills**
Positioning PSC
Placing robotic ports (appropriate depth)
Docking robotic ports to arms
Verifying adequate range of movement of robotic arms (avoiding conflict)
Switching robotic instrumentation during procedure
Adjusting SC for ergonomic use (height of arm rest, position of foot pedals, and so forth)
Use of master grips

Clutching (switching between instruments)
    Skills performed differently from Laparoscopic Cholecystectomy due to instrumentation
    differences

Use of electrocautery and bipolar sealing with foot pedals
Small space dissection with larger instruments
Knot tying technique

Box 3
Important Procedural Differences between Robotic and Laparoscopic Cholecystectomy

Step	Robotic Process	Robotic Subprocess	Median Robotic Time (min)	Median Laparoscopic Time (min)	Difficulty Difference
Preparation of operative field	Robot setup	PSC positioning	5 (3–7)	NA	H
		Docking of robotic arms	5 (3–6)	NA	H
		Verifying appropriate range of motion of robotic arms	14.5 (10–20)	NA	H
		Surgeon console setup	4 (2–5)	NA	=
Dissection of cystic duct	Retraction of gallbladder fundus	Grasping, retracting and locking gallbladder fundus	<30sec	NA- cannot lock instruments	E
	Exposure of cystic duct	Retraction of liver parenchyma with instrumentation	1 (0.5–4)	7.5 (7–8)	E
		Dissection of cystic duct within Calot's space	6 (3.5–8)	15.5 (13–18)	E
	Ligation of cystic duct	Knot tying of ligatures for cystic duct ligation	10 (5–13)	13 (12–14)	E
End of procedure	Removal of robotic instrumentation	Robot undocked from patient and PSC repositioned	4.5 (4–6)	NA	=

Abbreviations: = , no difference; H, harder than laparoscopy; E, easier than laparoscopy; NA, not applicable; PSC, patient side cart.

CHALLENGES FOR ROBOTIC SURGERY

While surgical robotics have helped human surgeons perform surgeries previously thought impossible, they do not come without cost and challenges. Even in human surgical communities, critics argue that the high cost of these systems limits accessibility to cutting-edge medical care for certain demographics and this will be the same for veterinary populations. Fortunately, multiple new robotic surgical options exist (Medicaroid, Medtronic, Stryker, Asensus, and so forth) which will improve availability and hopefully drive down costs. The ability to use the robot for certain surgeries does not mean it *should* be used and the associated added cost does not always appear to provide improved outcomes (refs). The operating room space required and the requirement for increased instrument inventory is also a consideration. Longer operative times due to the set up and docking of the instrumentation may lead to increased infection rates and could disqualify unstable patients due to safety concerns. For veterinary patients, one of the most important limitations is the size and length of the robotic ports and instruments. This feature currently limits their use in our smallest animals but ongoing work to improve human pediatric applications may benefit this patient cohort in the future.

SUMMARY

In conclusion, surgical robots are a remarkable fusion of cutting-edge technology and medical expertise that work together to provide surgeons and patients with unmatched precision, control, and visualization during minimally invasive surgeries. These devices have transformed the field of surgery, enabling complex procedures to be performed, and their use in veterinary medicine is already underway. While surgical robots do carry inherent challenges, research on when their use may be advantageous for our patients should be pursued so that we may usher in a new era of medical innovation and patient care.

CLINICS CARE POINTS

- Robotic instrumentations allows for improved surgical dexterity and surgeon ergonomics potentially increasing the variety of minimally invasive procedures performed in veterinary medicine.

- Robotic equipment and instrumentation, while sharing some similarities with traditional laparoscopic equipment, has many important differences, therefor proper training is vital before clinical cases are pursued.

- The procedures best suited for robotic interventions are those that require suturing, precise dissection and focus on one region of a body to minimize re-positioning of the robot during the procedure.

FUNDING

Cornell Affinitio-Stewart Grant for project titled Single Incision Robotic Cholecystectomy in a Cadaveris Dog Model.

SUPPLEMENTARY DATA

Supplementary data to this article can be found online at https://doi.org/10.1016/j.cvsm.2024.02.008.

REFERENCES

1. Young RF. Application of robotics to stereotactic neurosurgery. Neurol Res 1987; 9(2):123–8.
2. Drake JM, Joy M, Goldenberg A, et al. Computer- and robot-assisted resection of thalamic astrocytomas in children. Neurosurgery 1991;29(1):27–33.
3. National Museum of American History. Available at: https://americanhistory.si.edu/collections/nmah_1842522#:~:text=This%201989%20ROBODOC%20prototype%20is,of%20California%2C%20Davis%20Medical%20School. [Accessed 10 November 2023].
4. Cowley G. Introducing "Robodoc". A robot finds his calling–in the operating room. Newsweek 1992;120(21):86.
5. Bargar WL, Parise CA, Hankins A, et al. Fourteen Year Follow-Up of Randomized Clinical Trials of Active Robotic-Assisted Total Hip Arthroplasty. J Arthroplasty 2018;33(3):810–4.
6. Schulz AP, Seide K, Queitsch C, et al. Results of total hip replacement using the Robodoc surgical assistant system: clinical outcome and evaluation of complications for 97 procedures. Int J Med Robot 2007;3(4):301–6.
7. Jacofsky DJ, Allen M. Robotics in arthroplasty: a comprehensive review. J Arthroplasty 2016;31(10):2353–63.
8. Thiel DD, Winfield HN. Robotics in urology: past, present, and future. J Endourol 2008;22:825–30.
9. McGuinness LA, Prasad Rai B. Robotics in urology. Ann R Coll Surg Engl 2018; 100(6 sup):38–44.
10. Truong M, Kim JH, Scheib S, et al. Advantages of robotics in benign gynecologic surgery. Curr Opin Obstet Gynecol 2016;28:304–10.
11. Zhang TWD, Da L, Da L. Remote-controlled vascular interventional surgery robot. Int J Med Robotics Comput Assist Surg 2010;6:194–201.
12. Liu HH, Li LJ, Shi B, et al. Robotic surgical systems in maxillofacial surgery: a review. Int J Oral Sci 2017;9:63–73.
13. Navarrete-Arellano M. Robotic-assisted minimally invasive surgery in children. In: Kucuk S, editor. Latest developments in medical robotics systems, online. London: IntechOpen Ltd; 2021. p. 1–31. https://doi.org/10.5772/intechopen.96684.
14. Navarrete Arellano M, González FG. Robot-assisted laparoscopic and thoracoscopic surgery: prospective series of 186 pediatric surgeries. Front Pediatr 2019;7:200.
15. Liu Z, Zhang C, Ge S. Efficacy and safety of robotic-assisted versus median sternotomy for cardiac surgery: results from a university affiliated hospital. J Thorac Dis 2023;15(4):1861–71.
16. Rassweiler J, Frede T, Seemann O, et al. Telesurgical laparoscopic radical prostatectomy. Initial experience. Eur Urol 2001;40(1):75–83.
17. Queirós SF, Vilaça JL, Rodrigues NF, Neves SC, Teixeira PM, Correia-Pinto J. A laparoscopic surgery training interface. 2011 IEEE 1st International Conference on Serious Games and Applications for Health, SeGAH 2011. 1-7. 10.1109/SeGAH.2011.6165446. Accessed online November 15th, 2023.
18. Guru KA, Kuvshinoff BW, Pavlov-Shapiro S, et al. Impact of robotics and laparoscopy on surgical skills: A comparative study. J Am Coll Surg 2007;204(1):96–101.
19. Palep JH. Robotic assisted minimally invasive surgery. J Minim Access Surg 2009;5(1):1–7.
20. Gala RB, et al. Systematic Review of Robotic Surgery in Gynecology: Robotic Techniques Compared With Laparoscopy and Laparotomy.

21. Sarle R, Tewari A, Shrivastava A, et al. Surgical robotics and laparoscopic training drills. J Endourol 2004;18(1):63–7.

22. Kim HJ, Choi GS, Park JS, et al. Comparison of surgical skills in laparoscopic and robotic tasks between experienced surgeons and novices in laparoscopic surgery: an experimental study. Ann Coloproctol 2014;30(2):71–6.

23. Dixon F, Vitish-Sharma P, Khanna A, et al. Work-related musculoskeletal pain and discomfort in laparoscopic surgeons: an international multispecialty survey. Ann R Coll Surg Engl 2023;105(8):734–8.

24. Luger T, Bonsch R, Seibt R, et al. Intraoperative active and passive breaks during minimally invasive surgery influence upper extremity physical strain and physical stress response-A controlled, randomized cross-over, laboratory trial. Surg Endosc 2023;37(8):5975–88.

25. Armijo PR, Flores L, Pokala B, et al. Gender equity in ergonomics: does muscle effort in laparoscopic surgery differ between men and women? Surg Endosc 2022;36(1):396–401.

26. Jones ARE. A survey of work-related musculoskeletal disorders associated with performing laparoscopic veterinary surgery. Vet Surg 2020;49(Suppl 1):O15–20.

27. Hayashi MC, Sarri AJ, Pereira PASV, et al. Ergonomic risk assessment of surgeon's position during radical prostatectomy: Laparoscopic versus robotic approach. J Surg Oncol 2023;128(8):1453–8.

28. Krämer B, Neis F, Reisenauer C, et al. Save our surgeons (SOS) - an explorative comparison of surgeons' muscular and cardiovascular demands, posture, perceived workload and discomfort during robotic vs. laparoscopic surgery. Arch Gynecol Obstet 2023;307(3):849–62.

29. Shugaba A, Lambert JE, Bampouras TM, et al. Should all minimal access surgery be robot-assisted? a systematic review into the musculoskeletal and cognitive demands of laparoscopic and robot-assisted laparoscopic surgery. J Gastrointest Surg 2022;26(7):1520–30.

30. Intuitive Surgical, Inc. https://www.davincisurgerycommunity.com/systems_i_a. [Accessed 25 November 2023].

31. Bai F, Li M, Han J, et al. More work is needed on cost-utility analyses of robotic-assisted surgery. J Evid Based Med 2022;15(2):77–96.

32. Sadri H, Fung-Kee-Fung M, Shayegan B, et al. A systematic review of full economic evaluations of robotic-assisted surgery in thoracic and abdominopelvic procedures. J Robot Surg 2023;17(6):2671–85.

33. Yazici S, Tonyali S. Comparison of health-related quality of life changes in prostate cancer patients undergoing laparoscopic versus robotic-assisted laparoscopic radical prostatectomy: a systematic review. Urol J 2023;7707. https://doi.org/10.22037/uj.v20i.7707. Online ahead of print.

34. Wang J, Hu K, Wang Y, et al. Robot-assisted versus open radical prostatectomy: a systematic review and meta-analysis of prospective studies. J Robot Surg 2023;17(6):2617–31.

35. Bratilă E, Comandaşu D, Coroleucă C, et al. Robotic surgery a step forward in standardization of hysterectomy in patients with deep infiltrating endometriosis. Chirurgia (Bucur). 2023;118(1):73–87.

36. Bankar GR, Keoliya A. Robot-assisted surgery in gynecology. Cureus 2022;14(9):e29190.

37. Thigpen B, Koythong T, Guan X. Robotic-assisted laparoscopic ureterolysis for deep infiltrating endometriosis using indocyanine green under near-infrared fluorescence. J Minim Invasive Gynecol 2022;29(5):586–7.

38. Rahimi AO, Hsu CH, Maegawa F, et al. First assistant in bariatric surgery: a comparison between laparoscopic and robotic approaches: a 4-year analysis of the MBSAQIP database (2016-2019). Obes Surg 2023. https://doi.org/10.1007/s11695-023-06996-3. Online ahead of print.

39. Hilt L, Sherman B, Tan WH, et al. Bariatric Surgeon ergonomics: a comparison of laparoscopy and robotics. J Surg Res 2023;S0022-4804(23):00451. Online ahead of print.

40. Kauffels A, Reichert M, Sauerbier L, et al. Outcomes of totally robotic Roux-en-Y gastric bypass in patients with BMI ≥ 50 kg/m2: can the robot level out "traditional" risk factors? J Robot Surg 2023;17(6):2881–8.

41. Coleman K, Fellner AN, Guend H. Learning curve for robotic rectal cancer resection at a community-based teaching institution. J Robot Surg 2023;17(6):3005–12.

42. Calini G, Abdalla S, Abd El Aziz MA, et al. Ileocolic resection for Crohn's disease: robotic intracorporeal compared to laparoscopic extracorporeal anastomosis. J Robot Surg 2023;17(5):2157–66.

43. Peñafiel JAR, Valladares G, Amanda Cyntia Lima Fonseca Rodrigues 5 6, Avelino P, Amorim L, Teixeira L, Brandao G, Rosa F. Robotic-assisted versus laparoscopic incisional hernia repair: a systematic review and meta-analysis.

44. Bhatt H, Wei B. Comparison of laparoscopic vs. robotic paraesophageal hernia repair: a systematic review. J Thorac Dis 2023;15(3):1494–502.

45. Solaini L, Cavaliere D, Avanzolini A, et al. Robotic versus laparoscopic inguinal hernia repair: an updated systematic review and meta-analysis. J Robot Surg 2022;16(4):775–81.

46. Ma L, Luo H, Kou S, et al. Robotic versus laparoscopic surgery for hiatal hernia repair: a systematic literature review and meta-analysis. J Robot Surg 2023;17(5):1879–90.

47. Ghazal AH, Fozo ZA, Matar SG, et al. Robotic Versus Conventional Unicompartmental Knee Surgery: A Comprehensive Systematic Review and Meta-Analysis. Cureus 2023;15(10):e46681.

48. Fozo ZA, Ghazal AH, Hesham Gamal M, et al. A Systematic Review and Meta-Analysis of Conventional Versus Robotic-Assisted Total Knee Arthroplasty. Cureus 2023;15(10):e46845.

49. Gianduzzo T, Colombo JR, Haber GP, et al. Laser robotically assisted nerve sparing radical prostatectomy: a pilot study of technical feasibility in the canine model. BJU Int 2008;102:598–602.

50. Faber K, de Abreu AL, Ramos P, et al. Image-guided robot-assisted prostate ablation using water jet-hydro dissection: initial study of a novel technology forbenign prostatic hyperplasia. J Endourol 2015;29:63–9.

51. Okumura Y, Johnson SB, Bunch TJ, et al. A systematical analysis of in vivo contact forces on virtual catheter tip/tissue surface contact during cardiac mapping and intervention. J Cardiovasc Electrophysiol 2008;19:632–40.

52. Weinstein GS, O'malley BW Jr, Hockstein NG. Transoral robotic surgery: supraglottic laryngectomy in a canine model. Laryngoscope 2005;115:1315–9.

53. Boyd WD, Desai ND, Kiaii B, et al. A comparison of robot-assisted versus manually constructed endoscopic coronary anastomosis. Ann Thorac Surg 2000;70(3):839–42, discussion 842-3.

54. Kajiwara N, Kakihana M, Usuda J, et al. Training in robotic surgery using the da Vinci® surgical system for left pneumonectomy and lymph node dissection in an animal model. Ann Thorac Cardiovasc Surg 2011;17(5):446–53.

55. Jamet A, Hubert Maire J, Tran N, et al. Robot-assisted radical prostatectomy training: Description of a canine cadaveric model. Int J Med Robot 2022;18(3): e2381.
56. Schlake A, Dell'Oglio P, Devriendt N, et al. First robot-assisted radical prostatectomy in a client-owned Bernese mountain dog with prostatic adenocarcinoma. Vet Surg 2020;49:1458–66.
57. Buote N, Chalon A, Maire J, et al. Preliminary experience with robotic cholecystectomy illustrates feasibility in a canine cadaver model. Am J Vet Res 2023; 84(10):1–8.

Printed and bound by CPI Group (UK) Ltd, Croydon, CR0 4YY

03/10/2024

01040477-0009